CW01306102

THE ESSENTIAL GUIDE TO SWEDISH DEATH CLEANING

THE ESSENTIAL GUIDE TO SWEDISH DEATH CLEANING

HOW TO DECLUTTER AND ORGANIZE YOUR LIFE
WITH THE SWEDISH ART OF DÖSTÄDNING

INTENTIONAL LIVING

HANNA BENTSEN

Copyright © 2024 by Hanna Bentsen

All rights reserved. No part of this book may be reproduced, stored in a retrieval system, or transmitted in any form or by any means, electronic, mechanical, photocopying, recording, or otherwise, without the prior written permission of the publisher, Teilingen Press.

The information contained in this book is based on the author's personal experiences and research. While every effort has been made to ensure the accuracy of the information presented, the author and publisher cannot be held responsible for any errors or omissions.

This book is intended for general informational purposes only and is not a substitute for professional medical, legal, or financial advice. If you have specific questions about any medical, legal, or financial matters matters, you should consult with a qualified healthcare professional, attorney, or financial advisor.

Teilingen Press is not affiliated with any product or vendor mentioned in this book. The views expressed in this book are those of the author and do not necessarily reflect the views of Teilingen Press.

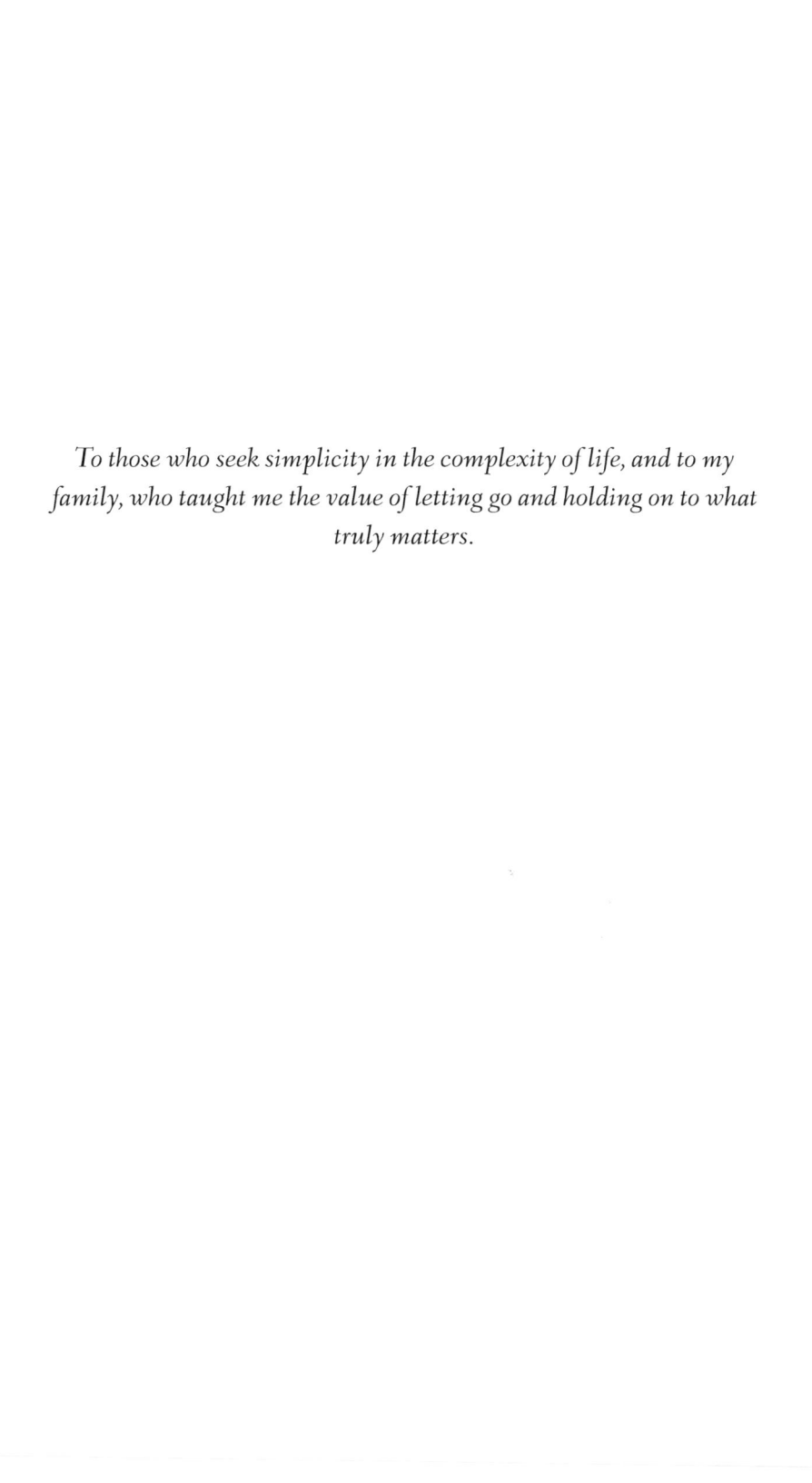

To those who seek simplicity in the complexity of life, and to my family, who taught me the value of letting go and holding on to what truly matters.

Out of clutter, find simplicity.

ALBERT EINSTEIN

CONTENTS

Introduction to Swedish Death Cleaning — xiii

1. PREPARING TO DEATH CLEAN — 1
   Creating a Plan and Timeline — 3
   Gathering Supplies and Resources — 4
   Communicating with Family and Friends — 6
   The Role of Forgiveness and Letting Go — 7
   Chapter Summary — 8

2. THE PROCESS OF DEATH CLEANING — 11
   Sorting Personal Belongings by Category — 12
   Dealing with Sentimental Items — 14
   Making Decisions: Keep, Gift, Donate, or Discard — 16
   Organizing and Storing What Remains — 18
   Chapter Summary — 20

3. TACKLING THE BIG STUFF — 21
   Electronics and Appliances — 22
   Books, Media, and Artwork — 24
   Clothing and Textiles — 25
   Papers, Documents, and Personal Records — 26
   Chapter Summary — 28

4. CLEANING AS YOU GO — 29
   Maintaining Order During the Process — 31
   Eco-Friendly Cleaning Practices — 32
   Dealing with Dust, Dirt, and Grime — 33
   Final Touches for a Refreshed Space — 35
   Chapter Summary — 36

5. MEMORIES AND MEMENTOS — 39
   Creating Keepsakes and Legacy Boxes — 41
   Digital Memories and Online Presence — 42

Sharing Stories with Family	44
Preserving Important Family History	45
Chapter Summary	47
6. THE EMOTIONAL JOURNEY	**49**
Attachment and Identity	50
Coping with Loss and Grief	52
Finding Joy in Letting Go	53
The Role of Reflection and Mindfulness	55
Chapter Summary	56
7. PRACTICAL MATTERS	**57**
Addressing Digital Assets and Passwords	59
Estate Planning and Wills	60
Funeral Wishes and Advanced Directives	62
Communicating Your Plans Clearly	64
Chapter Summary	65
8. THE ART OF GIVING	**67**
Choosing Meaningful Gifts for Loved Ones	67
Donations: Finding the Right Homes for Your Items	69
The Impact of Your Generosity	71
Gratitude and Reciprocity	72
Chapter Summary	73
9. OVERCOMING CHALLENGES	**75**
Dealing with Resistance from Others	77
Physical Limitations and Asking for Help	78
Staying Motivated and Keeping Momentum	80
Adapting the Process to Fit Your Needs	81
Chapter Summary	82
10. LIFE AFTER DEATH CLEANING	**85**
Continuing the Practices of Döstädning	88
Sharing Your Experience and Inspiring Others	89
The Ongoing Journey of Self-Discovery	91
Chapter Summary	92

The Lasting Impact of Swedish Death Cleaning   95

About the Author   103

INTRODUCTION TO SWEDISH DEATH CLEANING

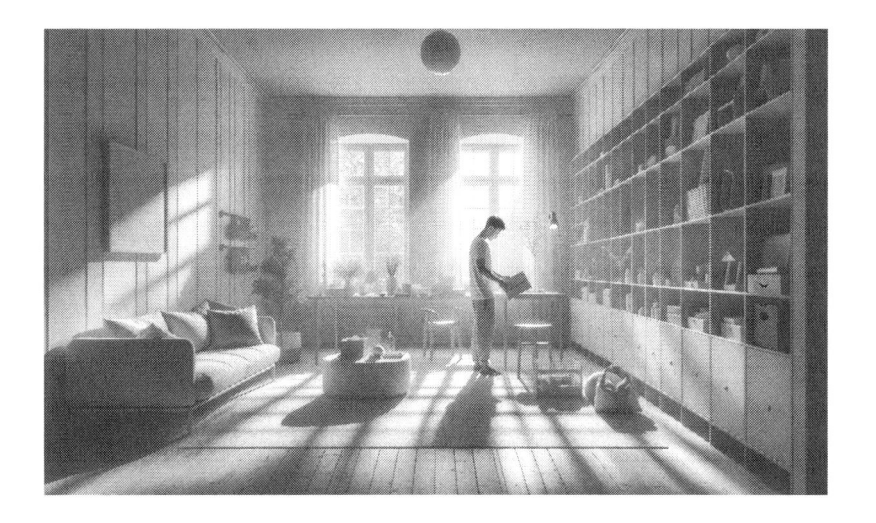

In the quiet corners of Swedish homes, a practice known as döstädning, or "death cleaning," has long been a part of life's natural rhythm. This philosophy is not merely about tidying up in the conventional sense; it is a deeper, more introspective process that intertwines with the Swedish cultural fabric. It is a deliberate and thoughtful act of sorting through one's belongings, not due to an imminent sense of one's mortality, but as a courtesy to those who remain and as a way to reflect on the memories of one's life.

The essence of döstädning lies in decluttering, simplifying, and organizing your material possessions to reduce the burden on loved ones who will inevitably have to deal with these items when you're no longer around. It is a systematic and reflective process that encourages individuals to examine their lives through the objects they have accumulated, discerning what truly holds value and what can be let go.

This philosophy is not a sad or morbid affair; instead, it is approached with a sense of pragmatism and care. It is about taking control of your belongings before they become a responsibility for someone else. The practice encourages people to keep only what they love and need, making their living spaces more manageable and their lives more focused.

At its core, döstädning is about legacy—what one chooses to leave behind for family and friends. It is an opportunity to pass on cherished possessions to loved ones, ensuring that each item carries a story or a memory rather than becoming an anonymous part of an estate sale. It is also a chance to relieve one's kin from the daunting task of sifting through decades of accumulation, which can be emotionally taxing and time-consuming.

The reflective nature of this cleaning process often leads to a profound sense of self-discovery and personal history. As individuals sift through their belongings, they may find themselves reminiscing, evaluating, and even coming to terms with different aspects of their lives. It is a way to acknowledge one's journey, celebrate achievements, reconcile with past regrets, and consciously curate the narrative one leaves behind.

In embracing the philosophy of döstädning, one also embraces a minimalist approach to living, which has been gaining traction in various cultures worldwide. This minimalist approach is not about

INTRODUCTION TO SWEDISH DEATH CLEANING

austerity or deprivation but about finding freedom and clarity by unburdening oneself from the excess that can often distract from life's true priorities.

As we delve further into the origins and cultural significance of Swedish death cleaning, we will uncover how this practice is a practical approach to household management and a deeply ingrained societal norm that reflects the Swedish ethos of simplicity, functionality, and thoughtfulness.

Origins and Cultural Significance

The pragmatic practice of Swedish death cleaning, or 'döstädning,' is a hybrid of the Swedish words for death ('dö') and cleaning ('städning'). This methodical approach to downsizing and decluttering one's possessions is deeply embedded in Swedish society, reflecting a thoughtful consideration for one's mortality and the impact it has on those left behind.

The origins of döstädning can be traced to a common-sense approach to living that values simplicity and practicality. In Sweden, there is a cultural inclination towards not burdening others with one's belongings after passing away. This ethos extends beyond cleaning and household management; it is a philosophy that intertwines with the Swedish concept of 'lagom,' which translates to 'just the right amount.' It is about finding a balance in life, not accumulating more than one needs, and keeping only those things that serve a purpose or bring joy.

Swedish death cleaning is not just a practice reserved for older people or those contemplating the twilight of their lives. It is a lifelong process that encourages individuals to regularly evaluate their possessions and consider each item's value and relevance. It is about creating a comfortable and orderly living space that reflects one's current life phase without excess material goods that can often lead to physical and emotional clutter.

The cultural significance of this practice extends beyond personal benefit. It is an act of kindness and consideration for family and friends. By systematically reducing one's belongings, individuals spare their loved ones the daunting task of sorting through a lifetime's worth of possessions. It is a final gesture of thoughtfulness, ensuring that the burden of material things does not overshadow the memories shared.

Moreover, Swedish death cleaning resonates with the concept of environmental consciousness. It encourages the repurposing, recycling, and thoughtful disposal of items, aligning with a broader commitment to sustainability and mindful consumption. This aspect of the practice embodies the importance of living responsibly with a consideration for the wider community and the environment.

The origins and cultural significance of Swedish death cleaning reflect a holistic approach to life and death. It is a practice that acknowledges the transient nature of existence and the importance of living a life that is both meaningful and considerate of the legacy one leaves behind. As we explore the interplay between mortality and materialism, we'll discover that döstädning is more than a cleaning method—it is a pathway to a more deliberate and intentional way of living.

Understanding Mortality and Materialism

When we ponder the inevitable journey each of us will take toward our own mortality, we come to realize that while our lives are transient, the material possessions we accumulate seem to outlive us, creating a silent legacy of our existence. This realization is at the heart of Swedish death cleaning, which encourages us to examine

INTRODUCTION TO SWEDISH DEATH CLEANING

our relationship with the objects we own and question what we wish to leave behind.

As we embark on this journey of decluttering with the end in mind, we are engaging in a process that is as much about introspection as it is about organization. It is a systematic approach that allows us to sift through the layers of our materialism to distinguish between what is truly valuable and what merely occupies space. This practice is not about eradicating memories or severing emotional ties but about curating them with intention and care.

The concept of materialism here is not to be frowned upon or dismissed as inherently negative. Our possessions, after all, often serve as tangible milestones of our life's journey—souvenirs from travels, gifts from loved ones, or heirlooms passed down through generations. Each item can hold a story, a memory, or a piece of our identity. However, in the context of Swedish death cleaning, we are prompted to consider the weight of these possessions, both literal and figurative, and how they might burden those we leave behind.

This reflective process is not hasty; it is methodical and can be intensely emotional. It asks us to confront our mortality and to make decisions about our belongings that reflect our final wishes. It is an act of kindness and consideration for those who will one day sift through what we've left, a way to ease their load and potentially spare them the arduous task of deciding what to keep, discard, and treasure.

In this light, Swedish death cleaning intertwines with the philosophical, urging us to ponder the impermanence of life and the permanence of the objects we leave in our wake. It is a deliberate, thoughtful process that aligns our external environment with our internal values, ensuring that our material possessions serve a purpose beyond our own tenure.

Next, we will explore how this practice brings peace of mind to the individual engaging in it and acts as a sincere gesture of love and respect for those who will carry on after us. The benefits of Swedish death cleaning extend beyond the individual, fostering a sense of continuity, connection, and care for the collective well-being of our loved ones and the memories we choose to leave with them.

Benefits of Death Cleaning for You and Your Loved Ones

In contemplating the inevitability of mortality, we uncover a heartfelt truth: the possessions we accumulate over a lifetime hold meaning both for us and for those we will one day leave behind. Swedish death cleaning is a compassionate and practical approach to addressing this reality. It is a process steeped in thoughtfulness, aiming to ease the burdens our material belongings might place on our loved ones after our passing.

The benefits of this practice are manifold. For the individual, death cleaning serves as a reflective exercise, a way to review one's life through the lens of physical objects. Each item we choose to keep or part with can reflect a cherished memory, a lesson learned, or a story we wish to pass on. This intentional sorting and decluttering can lead to a sense of peace and fulfillment, knowing that our material legacy will reflect our true values and the essence of what we hold dear.

Death cleaning can be a cathartic release from the often-unnoticed weight of possessions. As we sift through the layers of our material history, we may find ourselves unburdened by the past, free to live more fully in the present. The space we create in our homes can lead to a clearer mind and an environment that nurtures well-being. It is about making room not only in our closets and drawers but in our hearts and minds for new experiences and joys.

For our loved ones, the benefits of death cleaning are equally significant. In the wake of loss, sorting through a lifetime's worth of

INTRODUCTION TO SWEDISH DEATH CLEANING

belongings can be emotionally and physically overwhelming. By undertaking this process ourselves, we can spare our family and friends the daunting task of making difficult decisions about our possessions without our guidance. It is a final act of care and consideration, a way to ease their grief and to provide them with a curated collection of memories rather than a cluttered space to sort through.

Death cleaning can also serve as an opportunity for meaningful conversations with our loved ones about our possessions and the stories they carry. It allows us to share the significance of certain items, ensuring they are understood, appreciated, and preserved if we desire. It also opens a dialogue about our wishes, fostering understanding and reducing potential disputes over material things when we are no longer there to mediate.

In essence, Swedish death cleaning is about more than simply tidying up before we depart from this world; it is a deliberate and loving preparation for the inevitable transition we all must face. It is about taking control of our legacy, ensuring that what we leave behind is not a burden but a reflection of our life's narrative, carefully edited and thoughtfully arranged for those we love. As we embark on this journey, we set the stage for a process that is as much about celebrating life as it is about preparing for death.

Beginning Your Death Cleaning Journey

As we embark on the journey of Swedish death cleaning through the chapters of this book, it is essential to approach the process with a clear and prepared mindset. This approach to decluttering extends beyond tidying up; it is a thoughtful practice aimed at simplifying your life and leaving behind a considerate legacy. To set the stage for your death cleaning journey, we will delve into some practical steps to guide you through this reflective process.

Begin by acknowledging the scope of the task at hand. Death cleaning is not an overnight endeavor, nor is it a race. It is a gradual process that requires patience and perseverance. Start by setting realistic goals and timelines that resonate with your own circumstances. Whether you tackle one room at a time or categorize items by their emotional and functional value, the key is to proceed at a comfortable and manageable pace.

Next, gather the tools and materials to support you throughout this journey. Arm yourself with boxes, labels, and cleaning supplies. These will serve as helpful aids in your quest to sort, organize, and, if necessary, part with possessions. Consider also keeping a notebook or digital document to record your thoughts, decisions, and the stories behind certain items. This can be an invaluable resource for reflection and practicality, as it helps track your progress and the reasoning behind your choices.

As you prepare to dive into the physical aspects of death cleaning, take a moment to reflect on your intentions. Remind yourself of the benefits this process will bring to your own life and those of your loved ones. By reducing the burden of unnecessary belongings, you are crafting a clearer space and a more focused existence. You are also ensuring that your legacy is one of thoughtfulness and consideration rather than a daunting task for others to handle in your absence.

It is also important to consider the emotional journey that accompanies sorting a lifetime's worth of possessions. Some items will stir memories and emotions, and it is crucial to acknowledge and honor these feelings as they arise. Allow yourself moments of reminiscence and gratitude for the experiences and people that have shaped your life. However, remain steadfast in your resolve to make decisions that align with your ultimate goal of simplicity and mindfulness.

Lastly, do not hesitate to seek support. Whether it is the

companionship of a friend or family member during the sorting process or a professional's advice when appraising valuables, remember that you are not alone in this endeavor. Sharing the experience can lighten the load and provide a sense of camaraderie and shared purpose.

We will explore these moments of preparation in more detail in the next chapter. By properly preparing for the tasks ahead, you are setting yourself up for a thorough and meaningful decluttering journey. You may encounter challenges and emotional hurdles, but remember they are all part of the process, and the path you pave is one of clarity and generosity. Embrace the process with an open heart and a practical mind, and let the act of decluttering be an act of liberation and testament to a life well-lived.

Chapter Summary

- Döstädning, or Swedish death cleaning, is a reflective process of decluttering one's possessions as a courtesy to those who remain after one's passing.
- It is not a sad task but a pragmatic and caring act to control one's belongings and reduce the burden on loved ones.
- The practice is about legacy, allowing individuals to leave behind meaningful items with stories rather than anonymous clutter.
- It encourages a minimalist lifestyle, focusing on keeping only what is loved and needed. It is deeply rooted in Swedish culture.
- Swedish death cleaning reflects the Swedish ethos of simplicity and thoughtfulness, and it is not just for the elderly but a lifelong process.

- The practice is also environmentally conscious, promoting repurposing and recycling to align with sustainable living.
- It involves introspection and confronting one's mortality, curating possessions to reflect one's values, and easing the burden on loved ones.
- The process is gradual and requires preparation, patience, and support, ultimately aiming to leave a considerate and focused legacy.

1

PREPARING TO DEATH CLEAN

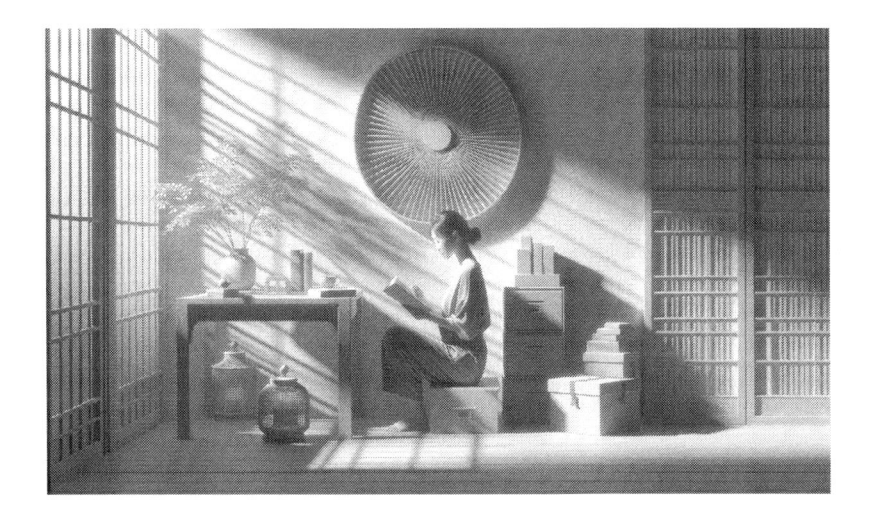

Embarking on the journey of Swedish death cleaning can be an intense and emotional process that requires a certain level of mental preparedness. It is a thoughtful and reflective act that involves sifting through a lifetime of possessions and deciding what truly matters.

Before diving into the practical aspects of decluttering, it is important to acknowledge the emotions that may surface. You may experience many feelings, from nostalgia to sadness, relief to anxiety. It is normal for memories to flood in as you handle various items, each with its own story and sentimental value. Allow yourself to sit with these emotions, to recognize and honor them. This process is as much about the physical items as it is about respecting your life and the memories you've created.

To prepare mentally and emotionally for death cleaning, start by reflecting on your intentions. Why have you decided to undertake this process? You may wish to simplify your life, provide a sense of order, or spare your family the task of sorting through your belongings. Clarifying your motivations will provide a sense of purpose and direction, making the process less daunting.

Next, consider the scope of what you will be dealing with. This is not a task to be rushed; it requires patience and thoughtfulness. It may be helpful to journal your thoughts and feelings as you go, providing an outlet for reflection and a record of your emotional journey.

Talking to your loved ones and sharing your intentions is also beneficial. Death cleaning is ultimately an act of kindness towards those you will one day leave behind. Discussing your plans can not only help you emotionally but can also provide comfort and understanding to your family and friends. They may offer support or share in the reminiscing, making the process a shared experience.

Remember, mental and emotional readiness is not about achieving a state of detachment or indifference. It is about approaching the task with a sense of peace and acceptance. It is about making deliberate choices that reflect your life, your values, and the legacy you wish to leave.

As you find yourself mentally and emotionally prepared, you may naturally progress toward creating a structured approach to your death cleaning journey. This involves establishing a plan and timeline to guide you through the practical steps of decluttering, ensuring the process is manageable and aligned with your personal goals.

Creating a Plan and Timeline

Once you've established the mental and emotional readiness to undertake the Swedish death cleaning process, it is time to focus on the practical aspects of this journey. Creating a plan and timeline is an important step that will provide structure and clarity to the task ahead.

Begin by assessing the scope of your possessions. Take a walk through your living space and make a mental inventory of the items that fill each room. Consider the furniture, the hidden items in closets and drawers, and even the keepsakes tucked away in attics or basements. This initial assessment will give you a sense of the magnitude of the task and help you estimate the time needed for each area.

Once you have a general overview, it's time to set realistic goals. Death cleaning is not a race; it is a deliberate process that may take weeks, months, or even years, depending on your circumstances and the volume of possessions to sort through. Decide on a timeline that feels comfortable for you. Some may prefer to dedicate a few hours each week, while others allocate entire days to the process.

As you create your timeline, consider the emotional weight of certain items. You may need to allocate more time to sort through personal mementos than you would for everyday household items. Be flexible and allow yourself the freedom to adjust your schedule as needed.

Next, break down your plan into manageable tasks. You might start with a particular room or category of items. For instance, beginning with clothing or books can provide a sense of accomplishment and momentum. As you progress, you can move on to more challenging categories.

It's also important to consider the logistics of disposing of items. Will you donate, sell, recycle, or discard the things you choose not to keep? Research local charities, second-hand shops, and recycling centers in advance. Knowing your options will make it easier to part with items when the time comes.

Lastly, keeping a record of your plan and timeline can be helpful. Whether a digital document or a handwritten journal, tracking your progress will help you stay on course and adjust your plan as necessary. It will also remind you of the work you have accomplished and the remaining steps.

By systematically planning your approach and setting a timeline that considers your emotional and physical needs, you can embark on a thoughtful and fulfilling journey toward a more intentional and unburdened life.

Gathering Supplies and Resources

It is essential to gather the right supplies and resources before delving into the task at hand. This preparation will facilitate a smoother transition through the various stages of decluttering and provide a sense of readiness and control, which can be particularly comforting.

To begin, you will need various sturdy boxes and bags for sorting items. These could come in different sizes to accommodate everything from books and papers to clothing and keepsakes. Labels or colored markers can help categorize these containers into groups such as 'keep,' 'donate,' 'recycle,' and 'throw-away.' This visual system will make organizing your belongings and tracking your progress easier.

Next, consider what cleaning supplies you may need for the

task. This could include cleaning cloths, dusters, sprays, and garbage bags. A clean and dust-free environment is conducive to thoughtful decision-making. Having a toolkit on hand for dismantling any furniture or fixtures you decide to part with is also practical.

In addition to physical supplies, you could also compile a list of resources that might be needed. This could include contact information for local charities that accept donations, recycling centers, and waste disposal services. You might also gather information on consignment shops, online marketplaces, or auction houses if you anticipate selling any items.

Documentation is another critical aspect of Swedish death cleaning. Ensure you have a filing system for important papers, such as wills, property deeds, and personal letters, which you may want to pass on or discuss with family members. A shredder might be necessary for securely disposing of sensitive documents that are no longer needed.

Lastly, it's beneficial to have a notebook or digital document to record your intentions for certain items, jot down memories or messages associated with particular belongings, and track your overall progress. This can be a reflective tool, allowing you to ponder the significance of the items in your life and the legacy you wish to leave.

Gathering these supplies and resources aims to create a supportive environment that will ease the physical and emotional workload of death cleaning. With everything in place, you can approach this task with a clear mind and a prepared heart, ready to make decisions that honor your life and your loved ones.

Communicating with Family and Friends

An essential step in the process is to open lines of communication with family and friends. Swedish death cleaning is a deeply personal and often emotional endeavor that affects the individual undertaking it and those around them. Therefore, it is important to approach this communication with sensitivity, clarity, and purpose.

Begin by setting aside a quiet time to talk with your loved ones. Explain the concept of Swedish death cleaning to them – the practice of mindfully organizing and reducing one's possessions to lessen the burden on others after passing. Emphasize that this is a proactive and considerate act, one that is done out of love and respect for those who will remain.

Express your desires and intentions clearly. Let them know that you are preparing for the future and seeking to create a more orderly and peaceful environment in the present. This is a time to share your thoughts on the significance of certain items, perhaps heirlooms or personal mementos, and to discuss who might appreciate or have use for them.

It's important to be receptive to their feelings and thoughts as well. They may have attachments to certain items or memories you are unaware of. This process can serve as a bridge to understanding. It can help in making decisions that honor the sentiments of all involved.

Encourage family members to ask questions and to express their preferences or concerns. Some may wish to claim certain items, while others may have practical suggestions for distributing or disposing of possessions. This dialogue can help prioritize what to keep, what to gift, and what to let go of.

Remember, this process is not about rushing or making hasty decisions. It is a gradual and thoughtful progression and also an opportunity to share stories, reminisce, and acknowledge the emotional weight that objects can carry. By involving your loved ones, you are preparing your estate and creating a space for collective reflection and understanding.

This communication can be seen as a gift in the spirit of Swedish death cleaning. It is a chance to ensure that your legacy is preserved in the way you wish and that the process of sorting through your life's collection is done with respect and consideration for those you love. It is a step towards peace of mind for you and your loved ones as you declutter with intention and grace.

The Role of Forgiveness and Letting Go

Before you begin sorting through your possessions, take a moment to stop and cultivate a mindset that embraces forgiveness and the art of letting go. The Swedish death cleaning process involves an emotional and psychological readiness to part with items intertwined with our life stories, but this is not always easy to do.

Forgiveness, in the context of death cleaning, is a multifaceted tool. It involves forgiving ourselves for the accumulation of belongings that we no longer need or may burden our loved ones after we are gone. It is a gentle acknowledgment that holding onto certain items out of guilt or obligation serves no one in the long run. We must also extend forgiveness to others who may have given us gifts or heirlooms that do not align with our current values or lifestyle. By releasing any feelings of resentment or obligation, we pave the way for a more thoughtful and intentional selection of what to keep and what to let go.

Letting go is a complementary process to forgiveness. It is the physical manifestation of our emotional release. As we sift through our belongings, we may encounter items that stir up memories of past conflicts, regrets, or unresolved issues. It is essential to recognize that holding onto these physical reminders does not change the past nor heal old wounds. Instead, by letting go of such items, we are making a conscious decision to move forward, to create space for new experiences and memories that are in harmony with who we are in the present.

The act of letting go also extends to our relationships. As we prepare for death cleaning, it is an opportune time to mend fences and express gratitude or apologies where needed. This does not mean we must keep every token of affection or every memento of a shared experience. Instead, it is about cherishing the essence of our relationships and allowing the physical items to be just that—items that do not define the depth or significance of our connections with others.

In practice, a few reflective exercises can facilitate forgiveness and letting go during the death cleaning process. Consider writing a letter to yourself or someone else, expressing the thoughts and feelings that arise as you handle each item. You do not need to send these letters; their purpose is to provide a private space for acknowledgment and release. Another method is to take a moment with each challenging item, thanking it for its role in your life, and then consciously deciding its fate—be it donation, recycling, or disposal.

Swedish death cleaning aims not to erase the past but to curate a legacy that reflects the most meaningful and loving aspects of our lives. By incorporating forgiveness and the practice of letting go, we can set ourselves up for a more meaningful and liberating death cleaning journey.

Chapter Summary

- Swedish death cleaning is a personal and emotional process that involves acknowledging emotions and reflecting on the life lived and memories created.
- Mental and emotional preparation for death cleaning includes understanding motivations, setting a purposeful direction, and patience.
- Communicating with family and friends about the process can provide emotional support and shared understanding.
- Creating a structured plan and timeline helps manage the decluttering process, considering the emotional weight of items.
- Gathering supplies like boxes, bags, cleaning materials, and a filing system for important documents is essential.
- The process aims to curate a meaningful legacy. Various strategies can help facilitate emotional release, including forgiving oneself for accumulated belongings and letting go of items that no longer serve a purpose.

2

THE PROCESS OF DEATH CLEANING

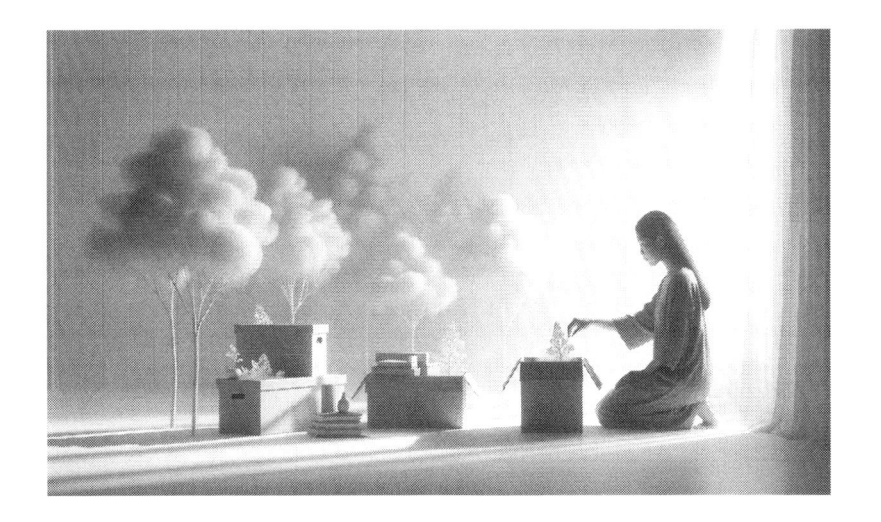

Having cultivated an intentional mindset and prepared yourself for the journey ahead, begin with the simplest tasks. This approach is practical and serves as a gentle introduction to the process, allowing you to ease into the more challenging aspects that may follow.

The first step is to identify items in your home that are the easiest to sort through. These objects often hold little sentimental value and are simply taking up space. You could begin with the miscellaneous drawer everyone has in their kitchen, filled with random utensils, takeout menus, and unclaimed keys. Or consider starting with your wardrobe, where clothes that no longer fit or have gone out of style can be the first to go. The goal is to build momentum, creating a sense of accomplishment to fuel your journey through the more sentimental items.

As you sort through these belongings, it's essential to remember the guiding principle of death cleaning: to minimize the burden on loved ones after one's passing. With each item you decide to part with, ask yourself if it will be valuable or useful to others. If not, it may be time to let it go. This process is not about discarding memories but about curating them. It's about making conscious decisions on what is truly important to keep and what can be released.

The systematic approach to starting with the simplest tasks also allows for reflection. With each item you handle, you're given the opportunity to reminisce and acknowledge its role in your life. This reflective practice is an integral part of Swedish death cleaning, as it helps in letting go of physical items and processing the memories and emotions attached to them.

Once the simplest tasks are underway and progress is visible, tackling the following category of belongings becomes easier. This gradual progression ensures that the process is manageable and that each decision is made with care and consideration. By starting simple, you lay a solid foundation for the more complex sorting that lies ahead.

Sorting Personal Belongings by Category

Having established a foundation by starting with the simplest tasks, we now transition into a more structured phase of the Swedish death cleaning process: sorting personal belongings by category.

This approach not only brings order to what may initially appear as an overwhelming task but also provides clarity and a sense of progress.

Begin by designating specific areas in your home for different categories. These categories include clothing, books, papers, household items, and personal mementos. Organizing items by category creates a visual and physical structure to guide you through the decluttering process.

When sorting clothing, consider the practicality and emotional value of each item. Ask yourself if the clothing is in good condition, has been worn recently, or holds significant sentimental value. Depending on their condition, clothes that are no longer needed or wanted can be donated, sold, or recycled.

Books, which often hold sentimental value, require a thoughtful approach. Reflect on which books have been meaningful to you and why. It may be helpful to consider whether these books would be of value or interest to others. If they are not, it might be time to let them go.

Papers can be one of the more daunting categories due to the sheer volume and the sensitive nature of the information they may contain. Start by discarding obvious items like outdated receipts, expired warranties, and old catalogs. Then, organize important documents such as legal papers, personal letters, and photographs, which may need to be kept or passed on to family members.

Household items encompass everything from kitchenware to decorative objects. Evaluate each item's usefulness and the likelihood of it being used by someone else. Items that are functional and in good condition are excellent candidates for donation or gifting.

Personal mementos are often the most challenging due to their emotional ties. While this category will be addressed in greater depth in the following section, it is important to approach these items with a balance of sentimentality and practicality. Consider which items genuinely enrich your life and which someone else might appreciate more.

Throughout this process, maintain a reflective mindset. Contemplate the life you have lived and the objects that have accompanied you along the way. This physical decluttering is also a thoughtful journey through your past, with a focus on creating a lighter future for yourself and your loved ones.

By categorizing your belongings, you create a manageable path forward in the death cleaning process. This structured approach allows you to address each category with focus and intention, making the task less overwhelming and more meaningful.

Dealing with Sentimental Items

As you sort through your belongings, you'll inevitably encounter the delicate task of dealing with sentimental items. Often brimming with personal history and emotional resonance, these objects can be the most challenging to address. They are the tangible manifestations of cherished memories, relationships, and experiences. In this process, we must tread with care, balancing respect for the past with the present and future practical necessities.

The first step in confronting sentimental items is acknowledging their emotional weight. Feeling strongly attached to personal mementos, such as photographs, letters, handmade gifts, or family heirlooms, is natural. These items often connect us with those we love and the moments that have shaped us. Recognizing the significance of these objects is crucial before any decisions are made about what to do with them.

Once we have honored the emotional significance of these items, it is time to reflect on their place in our lives moving forward. Ask yourself: Does this item still serve a purpose? Will it bring joy or utility to someone else? Is it something that I want to be part of my legacy? Reflection is a critical component of Swedish death cleaning and is especially pertinent to sentimental objects.

In this reflective process, it can be helpful to consider the concept of impermanence. Objects, much like life itself, are transient. Holding on to every item of sentimental value is neither feasible nor in keeping with the ethos of death cleaning, which is to simplify and unburden. It is about making room for the new physically and emotionally while still honoring the past.

One practical approach to managing sentimental items is to curate a selection of representative pieces. For example, instead of keeping every drawing your child ever made, you might choose a few that are particularly meaningful. This allows you to preserve the essence of your memories without being overwhelmed by volume.

Another approach is to digitize items where possible. Photographs, letters, and documents can be scanned and stored electronically. Digitizing saves physical space and ensures that these memories are preserved in a format that is less susceptible to decay over time.

For items unsuitable for digitization, consider whether they might find a second life with someone else. A piece of jewelry you no longer wear might bring a family member or friend joy. A collection of books could be donated to a library or school. In passing these items on, you give them a new purpose and extend their narrative beyond your own story.

When it comes to particularly challenging items that you cannot bear to part with but know you should, it may be helpful to involve a trusted friend or family member in the decision-making process. They can offer a fresh perspective and help you weigh the item's sentimental value against its practical considerations.

When dealing with sentimental items, giving yourself permission to let go is important. This does not mean discarding memories or relationships but consciously choosing what to carry forward. It is a process that requires time, patience, and self-compassion.

Making Decisions: Keep, Gift, Donate, or Discard

Having explored the delicate task of sorting through sentimental items, we now focus on the broader scope of belongings that populate our lives. The Swedish death cleaning process is not merely about decluttering; it is a thoughtful journey through your possessions, determining what truly matters and what can be let go. This phase—deciding whether to keep, gift, donate, or discard items—is perhaps the most critical step in the process.

To begin, establish a serene and undistracted environment. This will facilitate a clear and focused mindset, which is essential for making decisions you will be content with in the long run. Start with items that have less emotional weight. These are often easier to address and can help you build momentum and confidence in your decision-making abilities.

When considering each item, ask yourself a series of questions: When was the last time I used this? Does it bring me joy or serve a practical purpose? Could someone else benefit more from having this? Your answers will guide you toward one of four choices: keep, gift, donate, or discard.

Keep

Keep only those essential items that bring you happiness or have a designated purpose in your life. These are the things that you use regularly or that contribute positively to your daily existence. Be honest with yourself about what you truly need and value.

Gift

Gift items you no longer need but could have a meaningful second life with a family member, friend, or acquaintance. Gifting is a beautiful way to extend an item's life and share something of personal significance with others. It can be especially rewarding to pass on heirlooms or personal treasures to those who will appreciate and cherish them.

Donate

Donate items that are in good condition but do not hold significant personal value. There are many charities and organizations that can use clothing, books, furniture, and other goods to help those in need. Donating clears your space and contributes to the well-being of others and the wider community.

Discard

Throw away items that are broken, worn out, or otherwise no longer useful. This includes expired medicines, outdated electronics, and damaged goods. Disposing of these items responsibly, recycling where possible, and being mindful of the environment is essential.

Remember that Swedish death cleaning aims not to leave behind an empty home but to curate a space that reflects a well-lived life, free of unnecessary clutter. It's about making your surroundings as manageable as possible, both for you and for those who might inherit your space and belongings.

As you make these decisions, consider the practicalities of your current lifestyle and the legacy you wish to leave. Letting go can be liberating, and you craft a clearer, more intentional living space with each decision.

Once you have sifted through your belongings and made these decisions, the next step is to organize and store what remains to maintain the order and tranquility you've worked to achieve. This will ensure that your home is not only tidy but also that your cherished possessions are accessible and enjoyed in your daily life.

Organizing and Storing What Remains

Having navigated the emotionally charged waters of deciding which possessions to keep, gift, donate, or discard, you can now focus on the practicalities of organizing and storing the items that have earned their place in the 'keep' category. This is not a step to be overlooked in the Swedish death cleaning process, as it ensures that the retained items are accessible, well-maintained, and do not contribute to unnecessary clutter.

Begin by considering the space you have available. Be realistic about the volume of belongings you can comfortably store without overcrowding your living space. This might mean re-evaluating items if your available space is less than the volume of items you initially decided to keep. Remember, one of the goals of death cleaning is to create a serene and manageable environment for yourself.

Once you've confirmed that your kept items are in harmony with your space, focus on organizing them in a way that reflects their frequency of use and emotional value. Everyday items should be easily accessible, while those with sentimental value that are used less frequently can be stored in a way that protects them from dust and deterioration.

For instance, consider transparent storage containers for items you don't use daily but wish to keep visible. This allows you to appreciate these items without handling them, reducing the risk of physical damage. Labeling these containers can also be a thoughtful gesture, as it provides context and guidance for anyone handling your affairs in the future.

For documents and personal papers, create a filing system that is both logical and clearly labeled. This could include categories such as personal identification, property deeds, financial records, and sentimental letters. Ensuring these are well-ordered not only aids you in locating them when needed but also simplifies the process for your loved ones.

When storing clothing, prioritize garments that are seasonally appropriate and in good condition. Consider professional preservation methods if you have special attire that you no longer wear but wish to keep for sentimental reasons, such as a wedding dress or a military uniform. This could include acid-free boxes or vacuum-sealed bags that prevent aging and protect the fabric.

Finding a balance between aesthetics and practicality is essential for more oversized items like furniture or artwork. Suppose a piece of furniture is rarely used but holds significant sentimental value. Could it be repurposed or displayed differently to integrate it into your daily life? Artwork should be displayed in a manner that allows for enjoyment but also preserves its condition, away from direct sunlight and humidity.

Throughout this process, maintain a reflective mindset. Consider the memories and emotions attached to each item you organize and store. This journey allows you to revisit cherished moments and, in some cases, to let go of the past to embrace a more unburdened present.

Organizing and storing what remains after the death cleaning process is a deliberate act of curating your life's collection, tidying up your living space, and ensuring that what you leave behind is a true reflection of your legacy.

Chapter Summary

- The Swedish death cleaning process can begin with simple tasks, such as sorting through items with little sentimental value, to build momentum for tackling more sentimental belongings.
- Items can be sorted by category, including clothing, books, papers, household items, and personal mementos, with a focus on what to keep, gift, donate, or discard.
- Sentimental items should be addressed with care, considering their emotional significance and whether they should be kept as part of one's legacy or let go.
- Practical strategies for sentimental items include curating a selection of representative pieces, digitizing where possible, and involving others in the decision-making process.
- Decisions on belongings can be made by asking yourself if they bring joy, serve a purpose, or could benefit others, leading to keeping, gifting, donating, or discarding.
- When organizing and storing kept items, consider space availability, frequency of use, and emotional value, with a focus on accessibility and maintenance.
- The final goal is to create a serene and manageable living environment, with organized belongings that reflect a well-lived life and intentional legacy.

3

TACKLING THE BIG STUFF

In Swedish death cleaning, we confront the physical bulk of our existence: the furniture and oversized items that fill our spaces and, in many ways, define the backdrop of our lives. These pieces have supported us, literally and figuratively, and deciding their fate requires a blend of practicality and sentimentality.

As you approach the task of sorting through your furniture, it's essential to start with a clear plan. Begin by assessing each item for its current use and emotional value. Ask yourself: When was the last time this piece was used? Does it hold significant sentimental value, or is it simply occupying space? Be honest in your appraisal, as this will guide you in making thoughtful and decisive decisions.

Once you've evaluated your furniture, consider the options for each piece. Some items may be heirlooms or hold sentimental value for family members. Reach out to them to gauge their interest—this ensures that meaningful pieces are preserved within the family and helps in the letting-go process, knowing these items will continue to be cherished.

For furniture no longer needed or wanted, selling or donating can be a suitable path. Items can be sold through various channels, such as online marketplaces, consignment stores, or garage sales. When pricing, be realistic about the item's condition and market value. Remember, the goal is not necessarily to make a profit but to find the furniture a new home where it will be utilized and appreciated.

Donating is another avenue, particularly for items that may have low resale value but are still functional. Many charitable organizations welcome furniture donations, and some will even arrange for pick-up, easing the logistical burden. This option clears space and contributes to a good cause, aligning with the thoughtful ethos of death cleaning.

Disposal may be the only option for those pieces that are beyond repair or unsuitable for donation. However, it's essential to do so responsibly. Check with your local waste management services for guidelines on furniture disposal or recycling programs that may be available. Some materials, such as wood or metal, can be recycled, reducing the environmental impact of your clean-out.

Each item you part with has been a part of your story, and it's natural to feel a sense of loss or nostalgia. Allow yourself to experience these emotions, but also embrace the liberation that comes with making space—both physically and emotionally.

By systematically addressing the furniture and oversized items in your home, you create an environment that is more manageable and aligned with your current life stage. This thoughtful reduction of your belongings serves as a gift to your future self and loved ones, encapsulating the true spirit of Swedish death cleaning.

Electronics and Appliances

Now, we focus on the electronics and appliances that have served us throughout the years. Often brimming with modern convenience, these items can be surprisingly laden with memories and

THE ESSENTIAL GUIDE TO SWEDISH DEATH CLEANING

attachments. Yet, they demand a unique approach when it comes to decluttering.

Firstly, assess the electronics and appliances you possess. Consider their utility, condition, and the likelihood of their use in the future. Begin by gathering all such items from around your home into one area. This consolidation allows for a clearer perspective on what you have and what truly requires attention.

Reflect upon each item thoughtfully. That old radio might not have been turned on in years, but perhaps it was a gift from a dear friend. The blender, now gathering dust, might remind you of culinary adventures past. Acknowledge these memories and recognize that holding onto the physical item is not always necessary to preserve the sentiment.

Once you have decided which items will not accompany you further, consider their potential for a second life elsewhere. Electronics and appliances in good working order might find a welcome home with family members and friends or through donations to charity shops and organizations that specialize in providing essential items to those in need. This not only extends the useful life of the item but also contributes to a cycle of generosity and sustainability.

Responsible disposal is vital for items that are no longer functional or have become obsolete. Many electronics contain materials that are harmful to the environment if not handled correctly. Research local e-waste recycling programs or facilities that can ensure these items are disposed of in an environmentally friendly manner. Some manufacturers and retailers also offer take-back programs for their products, which can be a convenient option.

While sorting through your electronics and appliances, you may encounter cords, chargers, and accessories whose purpose has long been forgotten. These can quickly become clutter without us even realizing it. Gather these miscellaneous items and attempt to match them to their counterparts. Unpaired or unneeded items can be disposed of with the same care as electronics, often through the same recycling channels.

As you work through this section of death cleaning, remember to keep records of what you dispose of, especially if you discard items that may contain personal data. Wipe hard drives, perform factory resets on devices, and remove any SIM or memory cards. Your aim is to ensure that your personal information remains secure even as your possessions move on from your life.

Books, Media, and Artwork

Books, media, and artwork often hold significant emotional value and can tell the story of a lifetime of interests, passions, and memories. However, they must not be overlooked in the decluttering process.

Begin with books, which, for many, are not just reading material but treasured companions. Start by removing all the books from your shelves. Consider each one and ask yourself if it holds meaning for you or could be of value to someone else. It's important to be honest about whether each book will be reread or if it's time to pass it on. Consider donating books that no longer serve you to libraries, schools, or charity shops, where they can enrich the lives of others.

When it comes to media, such as DVDs, CDs, vinyl records, and even old cassettes or VHS tapes, reflect on the likelihood of revisiting these formats. With the digital age offering more compact and accessible ways to enjoy music and films, physical copies may be redundant. Digitize what you can't bear to part with, and find new homes for the rest. Some collectors and enthusiasts would cherish these items, and selling or donating them can give them a second life.

Artwork presents a unique challenge, as it often carries a strong emotional attachment and can be one of the more personal possessions one owns. Start by identifying the pieces you genuinely love and resonate with you or your family. If there are pieces that no longer speak to you, consider whether they might be appreciated by friends, family, or even local art schools. Remember, the aim is not to strip away all sentiment but to curate a meaningful and manageable collection.

By thoughtfully curating your collection of books, media, and artwork, you declutter your space and create a legacy of cherished memories that truly matter to you.

Clothing and Textiles

Clothing and textiles often hold a significant emotional value, as they are closely tied to personal identity and memories. However, they also represent a substantial volume of possessions that can burden those we leave behind if not thoughtfully curated.

Gather all clothing, linens, towels, and other textiles into one area. This allows you to assess what you own clearly. Handle each item individually, considering its usefulness, condition, and emotional significance. Ask yourself when you last wore or used it, and be honest about the likelihood of it being used in the future.

For clothing, start with items that are easiest to part with. This might include pieces that no longer fit, are out of style, or damaged beyond repair. Consider the practicality of the garment – for instance, heavy winter coats may not be necessary to keep if you live in a mild climate or have multiple similar items.

As you sort, create separate piles for different actions: one for items to keep, one for donations, one for recycling, and one for textiles that are too worn to be used by someone else and might serve better as rags or in textile recycling programs. Be mindful of the quality and condition of items intended for donation – charities often spend considerable resources disposing of items that cannot be used.

When it comes to sentimental pieces, such as a wedding dress or a hand-knitted sweater from a loved one, consider if someone in your circle would cherish it as much as you have. If not, think creatively about how to honor the memory it represents. A photograph of the item worn at a significant event, accompanied by a written memory, can preserve the sentiment without the physical object.

For linens and towels, apply the same criteria. Keep enough sets for your needs and a few for guests, but let go of excess. Remember, items in good condition can be a welcome donation to animal shelters or charitable organizations.

Throughout this process, take breaks when needed and allow yourself to reminisce about the passing of time that these items represent. Focus on lightening the load for your loved ones and ensuring that those you keep reflect a thoughtful and intentional life.

By the end of this exercise, you should have a more manageable collection of clothing and textiles that serve your current life and will not impose an undue burden on your loved ones in the future.

Papers, Documents, and Personal Records

As we delve into papers, documents, and personal records, we enter a territory often fraught with emotional weight and practical complexity. Often tucked away in drawers, cabinets, and boxes, these items can accumulate over a lifetime into a formidable collection. The Swedish death cleaning process encourages us to approach these personal archives with purpose and clarity, ensuring that what we leave behind is meaningful and manageable for those we love.

Begin by gathering all your documents in one place. This may seem daunting, but it is essential for taking stock of what you have. Once assembled, categorize your papers into three groups: essential, important, and dispensable.

Essential documents are those that are crucial for legal and personal identification purposes. These include birth certificates, marriage licenses, passports, wills, living wills, powers of attorney, and other legal documents necessary for settling your affairs. These should be kept in a secure but accessible location, and it is wise to inform a trusted person about where these documents can be found.

Important documents may not be critical for legal purposes but hold significant personal or financial value. This category includes property deeds, mortgage papers, vehicle titles, insurance policies, tax returns, and investment records. While these should also be kept secure, consider digitizing them to reduce physical clutter and ensure their preservation.

Dispensable documents are the most numerous and often challenging to sort through. These include old letters, greeting cards, photographs, receipts, manuals, and warranties. Reflect on the sentimental value of each item. Ask yourself if it brings you joy, will be meaningful to others, or serves a practical purpose. It may be time to let it go if it does not meet any of these criteria.

When it comes to personal letters and photographs, consider the feelings of others before discarding them. You might find that family members cherish certain items you consider trivial. Offer these to relatives or friends who may appreciate them. Shredding or recycling is often the most responsible way to dispose of papers that are no longer needed.

Take your time to consider the significance of each document, and do not rush the decision-making process. By systematically addressing the accumulation of papers, documents, and personal records, you are simplifying your own life and easing the burden on those who will one day sift through your memories and milestones.

Chapter Summary

- Heirlooms and sentimental items could be offered to family members, while unneeded items can be sold or donated.
- Dispose of unsalvageable furniture and more oversized items responsibly, considering recycling options for materials like wood or metal.
- Electronics and appliances should be evaluated for utility and condition, with working items donated and obsolete ones appropriately recycled.
- Books, media, and artwork require a balance of practicality and sentimentality, with meaningful items kept and others donated or sold.
- Clothing and textiles should be sorted, with excess and unworn items donated or recycled and sentimental pieces creatively preserved or passed on.
- Papers, documents, and personal records can be categorized as essential, important, or dispensable, with sensitive items securely stored or digitized.

4

CLEANING AS YOU GO

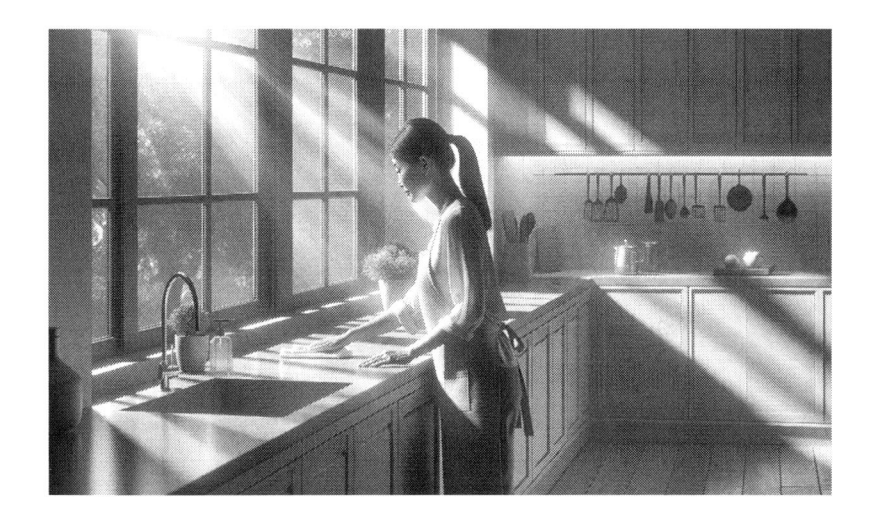

In the heart of Swedish death cleaning lies a principle that is as much about the present as it is about the future: the Clean Space Philosophy. This concept is a mindset, a way of living that simplifies the process of letting go and promotes a sense of tranquility in our daily lives.

The Clean Space Philosophy encourages you to approach cleaning not as a monumental task to be undertaken in the distant future but as a series of small, manageable actions integrated into everyday life. It is about creating and maintaining an environment that reflects the serenity we wish to leave behind. This philosophy is rooted in the understanding that our surroundings have the power to impact our well-being and that by curating our spaces thoughtfully, we can foster a sense of peace and order.

To embody this philosophy, we must first accept that every object in our possession carries emotional, physical, or psychological weight. By acknowledging this, we can assess our belongings more discerningly, asking ourselves whether each item serves a purpose or brings joy. If it does neither, it may be time to part with it. This is not to say that everything must go; it is about recognizing and holding onto what truly matters.

As we progress through our decluttering journey, it is essential to do so with intention. Each item we choose to keep should have a designated place within our home, a space where it belongs and contributes to the overall harmony of the environment. This deliberate placement of objects makes it easier to find what we need when we need it and creates a sense of order that is visually calming and mentally soothing.

The Clean Space Philosophy is about regular reflection and reassessment. As our lives evolve, so do our needs and preferences. What was once essential may no longer serve us, and what once brought happiness may no longer resonate. By periodically reviewing our possessions, we can ensure that our spaces remain aligned with our current selves rather than becoming time capsules of who we once were.

This philosophy is about cultivating a living environment that mirrors the clarity we seek in life. It is about recognizing that each day offers an opportunity to make choices that bring us closer to the essence of who we are and the legacy we wish to leave. By cleaning as we go, we not only ease the burden on ourselves and our loved ones in the future, but we also enhance the quality of our daily existence, creating a sanctuary that supports and reflects our journey through life.

Maintaining Order During the Process

As we progress further in our Swedish death cleaning journey, it is essential to recognize that the process is not simply a one-time event but a continuous practice of maintaining order. The philosophy of cleaning as you go is about instilling a sense of harmony and tranquility in your living space.

To maintain order during the process, remember to approach each task with mindfulness and intention. Set realistic goals for each cleaning session. Whether it's a single drawer, a closet, or a room, focus on that area and resist the urge to jump from one task to another. This targeted approach prevents feeling overwhelmed and keeps the process manageable.

As you sort through your belongings, categorize them into distinct piles or boxes and deal with each category promptly to avoid accumulating items that can lead to disorder over time. Assign the items you keep to a specific place in your home. This helps locate them when needed and discourages the piling up of unnecessary objects in the future. If you find items belonging to other family members or friends, set them aside so you can discuss their fate together. Swedish death cleaning is, after all, a considerate and communicative process.

During the cleaning sessions, take the time to clean the spaces that have been cleared. Wipe down shelves, vacuum or sweep the floors, and ensure that each item you return to its place is clean and in good condition. This habit contributes to the overall cleanliness of your home and the preservation of your belongings.

Be patient with yourself. Maintaining order is not about perfection; it's about progress. There will be days when you feel you've accomplished a lot and others when it seems you've barely made a dent. Acknowledge the effort you've put in and the steps you've taken towards a less cluttered and more intentional living space.

Lastly, remember to reflect on the emotional journey accompanying the physical act of cleaning. With each object you let go of, you're also releasing memories and attachments. Allow yourself to feel these emotions, reminisce, and come to terms with the impermanence of material possessions. This reflective process is integral to Swedish death cleaning, as it cleanses your home and provides clarity and peace of mind.

By maintaining order using these helpful pieces of advice, you are preparing for the eventualities of life and creating a serene environment that enhances your daily living. Swedish death cleaning can be an enriching and life-affirming process when done methodically and with intention.

Eco-Friendly Cleaning Practices

Another aspect to consider during the process is the environmental impact of our cleaning practices. The ethos of döstädning is also about minimizing our ecological footprint. In this spirit, let's explore eco-friendly cleaning practices that align with the thoughtful and purposeful approach of Swedish death cleaning.

Firstly, recognize the power of simplicity in cleaning agents. Commercial cleaning products often contain chemicals that can harm our health and the environment. Instead, consider natural alternatives like white vinegar, baking soda, and lemon juice, which are effective, non-toxic, and biodegradable. These simple ingredients can tackle various cleaning tasks, from descaling a kettle to freshening up laundry.

Use reusable cloths and sponges rather than disposable paper towels when scrubbing and wiping surfaces. Microfiber cloths, for instance, are highly absorbent and can be washed and reused countless times, reducing waste. If you prefer something more natural, consider bamboo or organic cotton cloths.

In decluttering, you might come across old t-shirts or towels. Rather than discarding them, repurpose them into cleaning rags. This extends the life of these materials and reduces the need to purchase new cleaning cloths.

For those items that require a deeper clean, such as carpets or upholstered furniture, look for eco-friendly professional services that use non-toxic cleaning methods. Alternatively, renting or investing in a steam cleaner for personal use can be a chemical-free way to refresh these items without the environmental toll of conventional cleaning solutions.

Consider the most environmentally responsible methods when disposing of items that no longer serve a purpose in your life. Recycle what you can, donate items still in good condition, and responsibly discard electronics and hazardous materials according to local regulations.

Lastly, remember that the goal is not only to leave behind a tidy and considerate legacy but also to do so in a way that honors the environment. By integrating eco-friendly cleaning practices into this process, you contribute to a healthier planet for current and future generations.

Dealing with Dust, Dirt, and Grime

The Swedish death cleaning philosophy extends beyond merely sorting and discarding items. It encompasses the meticulous care of our living spaces, ensuring they remain clean, orderly, and pleasant. As we adopt the principles of 'döstädning,' we should also focus on the persistent adversaries of cleanliness: dust, dirt, and grime.

These elements are reminders of the passage of time and the accumulation of life's residues. Addressing them is not a sporadic battle but a continuous process. It is about maintaining an environment that reflects our respect for our possessions and the eventual ease of transition for those we leave behind.

To deal with dust, begin with the high surfaces and work your way down. Use a microfiber cloth or a duster with an extendable handle to reach the tops of bookshelves, picture frames, and light fixtures. This method ensures that any dislodged particles will ultimately find their way to the floor, where they can be swept or vacuumed away in the final cleaning stages.

When confronting dirt and grime, especially in high-traffic areas or places where spills and stains are common, acting swiftly and with the appropriate cleaning agents is essential. For hard surfaces, a mixture of warm water and mild dish soap can be effective, while a baking soda paste might be necessary for more stubborn grime. Always test a small, inconspicuous area first to ensure the cleaning solution does not damage the surface.

In the case of upholstery and fabrics, vacuuming regularly is crucial to prevent the embedding of dirt and dust. For stains, use a cleaner suitable for the fabric type and blot gently, avoiding harsh scrubbing that can damage the fibers.

Throughout this process, take a moment to reflect on the items you are cleaning. Each object has a story and a connection to your life. As you wipe away the dust and grime, you are also reaffirming your decisions about what to keep and what to let go. This cleaning becomes a physical manifestation of our internal contemplation, an organized practice that cleans our homes and clears our minds.

Integrating these cleaning practices into our routine ensures that our living spaces remain decluttered and reflect a well-loved life. It is a gift of consideration to ourselves and those who will one day be responsible for our cherished belongings. Maintaining cleanliness is an act of kindness that will echo into the future.

Final Touches for a Refreshed Space

Having addressed the removal of dust, dirt, and grime, we can now turn our attention to the final touches that transform a clean space into a refreshed and harmonious environment. This step is as much about cleanliness as it is about creating a sense of peace and harmony that can be felt by anyone who enters the space.

Begin by stepping back and surveying the room. After thoroughly cleaning, the space should already feel more open and inviting. However, the final touches are about fine-tuning the area to ensure it feels truly finished and welcoming. This involves a few key steps that are often overlooked but essential for achieving the desired effect.

Firstly, consider the placement of furniture and objects. During the cleaning process, items may have been moved around to allow for a more thorough job. Now is the time to thoughtfully rearrange these pieces to optimize the flow and functionality of the room. In the spirit of döstädning, this may also be an opportunity to reassess the necessity of certain items. If something no longer serves a purpose or brings joy, it may be time to let it go.

Next, focus on the more minor details. Polish mirrors and glass surfaces to a streak-free shine, as these can often show the remnants of cleaning products if not properly attended to. Fluff cushions and straighten throws to give a lived-in yet tidy appearance to seating areas. These small actions contribute significantly to the overall sense of order and comfort.

Lighting plays a pivotal role in the ambiance of a room. Adjust the window treatments to allow natural light to filter in, enhancing the freshness of the space. If the room is used in the evening, ensure the lighting is warm and inviting. A well-placed lamp or a dimmer switch can make all the difference in creating a cozy atmosphere.

Finally, add a personal touch that signifies the completion of the cleaning process. This could be a fresh bouquet of flowers placed in a vase, a scented candle, or a piece of art with special meaning. These elements serve as a reminder of the care and intention put into the cleaning process and the importance of maintaining a space that reflects the best aspects of one's life.

These final touches are about more than just aesthetics; they reaffirm the values and memories we wish to preserve and pass on. By methodically and reflectively approaching this last stage, we not only create a space that is clean and organized but also one that will bring joy to our everyday lives.

Chapter Summary

- The Clean Space Philosophy emphasizes living with tranquility by integrating small cleaning actions into daily life.
- Regular reflection and reassessment of belongings are encouraged to align living spaces with current needs and preferences.
- Maintaining order during cleaning involves setting realistic goals, categorizing items, and cleaning spaces as they are cleared.
- Eco-friendly cleaning practices are recommended, such as using natural cleaning agents and repurposing old materials for cleaning rags.
- Dust, dirt, and grime should be addressed methodically, with appropriate cleaning agents and techniques for different surfaces.

- Final touches in the cleaning process involve thoughtful placement of furniture, polishing surfaces, optimizing lighting, and adding personal touches.
- Swedish death cleaning is a continuous process that not only prepares for the future but also creates a serene environment for the present.

5

MEMORIES AND MEMENTOS

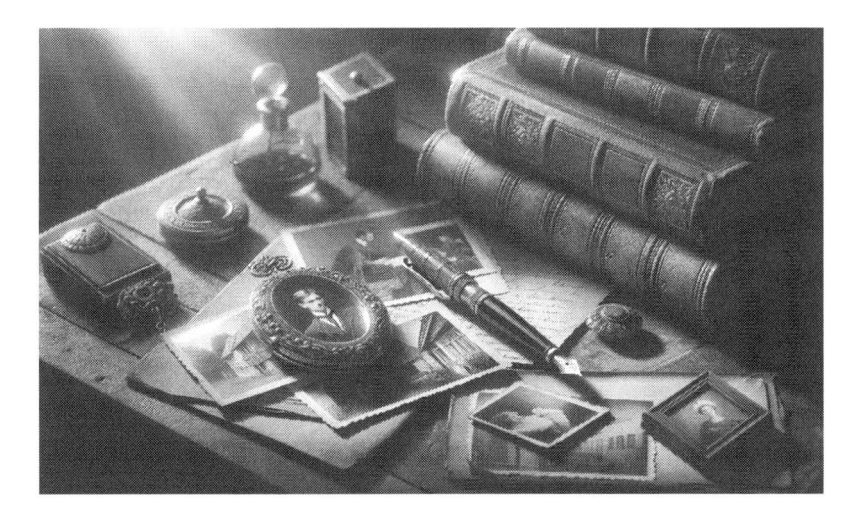

As we find ourselves sifting through the tangible remnants of our lives—photographs, letters, and keepsakes— each item can evoke a spectrum of emotions, from joy to sorrow, nostalgia to resolve. In curating your life story through these mementos, you are not only reflecting on the past but also shaping the legacy you wish to leave behind.

Selecting which memories to preserve and which to let go of is akin to editing a manuscript of your life. It requires a discerning eye and a thoughtful heart. Here is some guidance to help you sort through these possessions carefully and intentionally.

Begin by gathering all your mementos in one place, creating a physical timeline of your life. As you examine each item, ask yourself: Does this object still hold meaning? Is it tied to a person or an event significant to me or my loved ones? Will it bring joy or comfort to those I leave behind?

It is important to recognize that not all possessions are created equal in emotional value. Some items may be intrinsically linked to pivotal moments or relationships. In contrast, others, upon reflection, may be mere placeholders for memories that reside securely in your mind. It is the former that merit a place in your curated collection.

As you make these decisions, consider the stories these objects tell. A well-worn recipe card, annotated with notes and stains, tells a tale of family gatherings and shared meals. A collection of postcards may map out a lifetime of travels and adventures. These items are all part of your life story, a narrative you will pass on.

In this process, it is also essential to be mindful of the quantity of items you choose to keep. A life story distilled into a few cherished possessions can often speak louder than a volume of cluttered memories. This is not to say that you should strip your history to the bare bones, but rather to select those pieces that best represent the essence of your journey.

Remember, too, that this curation is not a solitary task. Engage with family and friends, sharing the stories behind your treasures. Their insights may help you see the value in items you overlooked, or they may lovingly relieve you of the burden of objects that hold more meaning for them than for you.

Ultimately, the goal of curating your life story is not to create a shrine to oneself but to craft a thoughtful collection that honors your past, brings peace in the present, and will be cherished by those who continue your story into the future.

Creating Keepsakes and Legacy Boxes

As we sift through our personal treasures, we may wonder how best to preserve these stories for future generations. This is where the concept of creating keepsakes and legacy boxes comes into play.

A keepsake is an item that holds personal value and evokes memories of a particular time, person, or event. It is something to be cherished and passed down through the family as a token of remembrance. On the other hand, a legacy box is a carefully curated collection of such keepsakes thoughtfully assembled to convey a narrative of one's life journey.

You may wish to create a legacy box for some of your most sentimental items. Selecting items for a legacy box requires a reflective and systematic approach. Begin by choosing a container that feels appropriate for the treasures it will hold. This could be a beautifully crafted wooden box, a sturdy archival storage box, or even a simple yet elegant cardboard box. The container itself can be a part of the legacy, reflecting the aesthetic preferences of its assembler.

As you decide on the contents, consider the stories each item tells. A legacy box is more than just a repository for things; it is a vessel for stories, a way to communicate values, experiences, and the essence of who you are. Include items that have a narrative quality: letters, photographs, a cherished book, or a piece of jewelry that has been passed down through generations. Each of these items should serve as a chapter in the story of your life.

You could include a personal note or a descriptive label with each item. This narrative can explain the significance of the object, the context in which it was received or used, and why it has been chosen to be part of the legacy. These descriptions will provide clarity and meaning for those who will one day sift through these memories.

Balancing emotional value with practical considerations is vital when creating keepsakes and legacy boxes. Be selective and avoid overfilling the box. The goal is to distill a life's worth of memories into a collection that is meaningful, manageable, and, most importantly, reflective of yourself.

As you curate these items, you may find yourself reminiscing and reflecting on the life you've led. This process is about leaving a legacy for others and reviewing and appreciating the life you have lived. It is a chance to acknowledge your journey, the people who have been part of it, and the moments that have defined you.

Creating keepsakes and legacy boxes is an act of love, a final gift to your loved ones, and a way to ensure that your story is told and remembered.

Digital Memories and Online Presence

In the modern age, the concept of mementos extends beyond the tangible. As we continue our journey of reflection and self-discovery, we must also consider the digital footprint we leave behind. Digital memories and online presence form a significant part of our legacy, and managing them can be as meaningful as handling physical belongings.

Our digital lives are composed of photographs, videos, social media profiles, blogs, and email accounts, each holding pieces of our narratives. These virtual keepsakes are often overlooked during the decluttering process. Yet, they require our attention to ensure that our digital legacy aligns with our wishes and provides a clear, curated story, free from clutter for those we leave behind.

Begin by taking inventory of your digital assets. List all the platforms and accounts where you have a presence. This includes social media profiles, cloud storage services, email accounts, and any websites or blogs you own. Reflect on what each of these digital spaces represents about you and how they contribute to the story you wish to tell.

For social media accounts, consider downloading a copy of your data, which is often a feature offered by the platforms. This lets you keep a personal archive of your interactions, photos, and posts. Once you have this archive, you might deactivate certain profiles or leave instructions on handling them when you are no longer around. Some platforms have legacy contact options, enabling a trusted person to manage your account after you pass away.

Photographs and videos stored in the cloud or digital devices are precious memories that can be shared with loved ones. Organize these by creating folders for different periods or events and label them clearly. You might also consider transferring these to a dedicated external hard drive or creating shared online albums for family and friends to access.

Email accounts often contain a mix of important documents and casual correspondence. Sift through your emails, deleting what is no longer necessary and organizing the rest into folders. It's also wise to leave instructions on handling your email accounts, including login information, as part of your digital estate planning.

For blogs and personal websites, decide if you want them to remain online as a record of your interests and thoughts. If so, ensure that the hosting fees are taken care of and that someone knows how to manage the content in your absence.

By taking these steps, you ensure that your digital memories and online presence are preserved and presented in a way that honors your life story. Just as with physical items, the goal is to leave behind a digital space that is organized, meaningful, and reflective of your life. This thoughtful approach to your digital legacy is a gift to those who will cherish your memory long after you're gone.

Sharing Stories with Family

Sharing stories with family is a crucial step in this journey. It breathes life into cherished objects and ensures their legacy continues even as we consider letting them go. This stage of the process is less about the physical act of decluttering and more about the emotional resonance of the items we hold dear.

When we engage with our family members in the storytelling of our possessions, we do more than recount the past; we create a bridge to the future. Each item, from a simple handwritten letter to a well-worn piece of jewelry, carries a narrative that, when shared, can offer comfort, instill values, and even impart wisdom. Through these shared narratives, our belongings transcend their material form and become part of our family's collective memory.

When you undertake this process, you might want to gather your family in a comfortable setting, free from the distractions of daily life. Approach the conversation with a sense of openness and invite your loved ones to ask questions. As you pick up each memento, allow yourself to delve into the memories it conjures. Describe the context in which the item was received or purchased, the people associated with it, and the reasons it has been significant in your life.

It is important to be reflective and honest during these exchanges. Some stories may evoke laughter, while others might summon tears. Both reactions are valuable and contribute to the richness of your history. Encourage family members to share their recollections and associations with the items. This can be particularly enlightening, as the same object may hold different meanings for different people.

As you share these stories, consider the practical aspects of Swedish death cleaning. Discuss with your family who might like to inherit certain items. This is an opportunity to match possessions with those who will truly appreciate and honor their history. It is also a chance to let go of things that, while once meaningful, no longer serve a purpose or bring joy.

Sometimes, while the physical item is not needed, the story behind it is precious. In these instances, documenting the narrative can be a powerful alternative to keeping the object. Write down the tales or record them, creating a lasting record that can be revisited and cherished for future generations.

Sharing stories with family is part of an ongoing conversation. It is a process that can be revisited as you continue to sort through your belongings and as your family's dynamics evolve. Doing this ensures that the essence of your memories is preserved, even if you make the thoughtful decision to part with the physical mementos.

Preserving Important Family History

Döstädning allows us to confront the tangible fragments of our past—those objects that carry the weight of our personal and family history. As we sift through the layers of belongings, we often unearth mementos that are more than mere objects; they are the keepers of stories, the physical manifestations of our lineage and legacy. Preserving these important pieces of family history is both a gift to our descendants and a way to honor the lives that have preceded our own.

The process begins with discernment. Certain pieces stand out as irreplaceable conduits to the past among the myriad of items that fill our homes. These may include photographs, handwritten letters, diaries, military medals, or even a simple recipe card in a loved one's handwriting. Each of these items holds a thread that, when woven together, creates the rich narrative of a family's history.

To preserve these treasures, we must first ensure their physical longevity. This involves practical measures such as storing paper items in acid-free sleeves, keeping photographs out of direct sunlight, and protecting delicate textiles from the ravages of time and environment. It is also advisable to digitize these items, creating electronic copies that can be shared and saved without physical deterioration.

But preservation goes beyond mere conservation of the object; it involves safeguarding the stories they represent. Take the time to document the history behind each memento. Who did this belong to? What is the story of its significance? Recording these details can be as simple as writing a note to accompany the item or as elaborate as creating a digital archive with narratives, images, and scanned documents.

Sharing these preserved items with family members can be a deeply meaningful experience. It provides an opportunity to connect with relatives over shared heritage and to pass on the stories of ancestors to younger generations. Consider creating a family history box or scrapbook that can be added to over time and passed down through the generations.

In the spirit of döstädning, it is vital to be selective. Not every item needs to be kept for posterity. Choose those that truly encapsulate the essence of your family's story and let go of the rest with gratitude for their role in your journey. This selective process not only eases the burden on those who will one day sift through our possessions but also highlights the most significant chapters of our family narrative.

Preserving important family history is a balancing act between honoring the past and embracing the impermanence of life. It is a thoughtful process that allows us to curate a legacy, ensuring that the stories and memories that shape us are not lost to time but are held close, ready to be retold and cherished by the generations to come.

Chapter Summary

- Sorting through tangible mementos like photos and letters is like editing a life story, requiring a discerning eye to choose items with emotional value and significance to oneself and loved ones.
- Not all possessions hold the same emotional value; it's essential to curate a collection that truly represents one's life journey.
- Creating keepsakes and legacy boxes involves selecting meaningful items that tell the story of one's life to be cherished by future generations.
- Engaging family and friends in the process can provide different perspectives and help determine the significance of items.
- Digital memories, such as social media profiles and online photos, are also part of one's legacy and should be curated with care and intention.
- Sharing stories with family about cherished items can create a bridge to the future and ensure the legacy of these objects continues.
- Preserving important family history involves being selective with items, ensuring their physical and narrative preservation, and sharing them with family.

6

THE EMOTIONAL JOURNEY

Throughout the process, you must be prepared for the emotional ebbs and flows that accompany the sorting and letting go of a lifetime's accumulation of belongings. It is a unique and personal journey that often brings to the surface various memories and feelings intertwined with the objects we have cherished.

As you navigate through the highs and lows of this journey, acknowledge that each item you touch may evoke a spectrum of emotions. The highs can be moments of rediscovery and joy as you unearth forgotten photographs that bring back the laughter of a summer long past or a treasured gift from a dear friend that reminds you of a bond that time or distance could erode. These moments buoy your spirits and remind you of the love and experiences that have colored your life.

Conversely, the lows can manifest as a sense of loss or grief. Parting with items can feel like saying goodbye to a part of yourself, a tangible connection to your past that you are not yet ready to sever. It may be a piece of furniture that has been the silent witness to your family's history or a collection of letters that speak of a younger self with dreams and aspirations now transformed by time.

Letting go can sometimes feel like you're erasing these chapters of your life.

Approach these emotional lows with compassion and patience. Allow yourself to feel the weight of these emotions, to sit with the sadness or the longing that may arise. It is a natural response to the closing of a chapter, an integral part of acknowledging and honoring your life's journey.

There is also an opportunity for growth and self-reflection in this emotional landscape. With each decision to keep or part with an item, you reaffirm your values and priorities. You are distilling the essence of your life story, deciding what is truly significant and what can be released. This discernment is empowering, as it clarifies what you wish to leave behind as your legacy.

Remember, Swedish death cleaning is not just about the physical act of decluttering but also about the emotional reckoning with one's mortality and the impermanence of life. It is a chance to confront the reality that we will all be a memory one day. In this confrontation, a great opportunity exists to shape that memory with intention and thoughtfulness.

As you continue on this journey, take solace in the knowledge that the emotional highs and lows reflect a life fully lived, the connections you've made, and the impact you've had on the world around you. Embrace the process as a meaningful ritual, an act of caring for those you will one day leave behind.

Attachment and Identity

Throughout the cleaning process, we confront the physical accumulation of a lifetime and the intricate web of attachment and identity that our possessions represent. This practice, while pragmatic in its approach to decluttering, is deeply interwoven with the emotional fabric of our being. It is a poignant reminder that the items we gather are more than mere objects; they are the silent narrators of our personal history, the tangible touchstones of our identity.

As we sift through the layers of belongings, we often stumble upon items that are heavy with memory and meaning. A simple piece of jewelry may carry the weight of a thousand moments, a book may open to a page that once offered solace, and a photograph may freeze time in a frame, holding faces and places that have long since changed. These are the artifacts of our existence, the physical manifestations of our joys, sorrows, achievements, and relationships.

Therefore, the act of letting go becomes more than a practical tidying up; it is a reflective journey through the chapters of one's life. Each decision to keep or discard an item is a negotiation with the past, a dialogue between the person we once were and the one we have become. It requires us to ask ourselves difficult questions about what is truly important and what legacy we wish to leave behind.

In this delicate dance of detachment, we may find that our sense of self is not diminished but rather distilled. By releasing the physical anchors of our past, we grant ourselves the freedom to redefine our identity. We learn that while objects can signify love, achievement, or heritage, they do not encapsulate the entirety of our existence. Our worth is not measured by the things we own but by the experiences we've had, the relationships we've nurtured, and the growth we've fostered within ourselves.

Swedish death cleaning, then, is as much an inward journey as it is a physical undertaking. It is an opportunity to reassess and reaffirm our values, acknowledge the impermanence of material possessions, and embrace the essence of who we are beyond the clutter. As we prepare our belongings for their eventual parting from us, we are also preparing ourselves for a future unburdened by the unnecessary. In this future, our identity is not tied to the objects we leave behind but to the memories and love we've shared.

Coping with Loss and Grief

As we sift through our belongings, we are inevitably faced with the memories and sentiments attached to them, and this can lead us into the depths of loss and grief. It is a natural part of the journey, requiring both acknowledgment and navigation with care.

Loss and grief are not solely the domain of those who have passed. They are also experienced by the living, who must grapple with the void left behind. In the context of death cleaning, these emotions can surface as we handle items that once belonged to loved ones or as we contemplate our mortality and the legacy we wish to leave.

Sorting personal belongings can trigger grief, as each item might evoke a memory, moment, or shared experience. It is not uncommon to feel a wave of sadness when holding a garment that still carries the scent of a departed loved one or when stumbling upon a handwritten note that speaks from the past. These tangible pieces of history serve as conduits to our emotions, and it is essential to honor these feelings rather than suppress them.

To cope with the grief that may arise during death cleaning, it is helpful to approach the task with a sense of ritual and respect. Allow yourself moments of reflection when they are needed. It is okay to pause, remember, and feel the full weight of what these objects represent. Some may find solace in sharing stories about the items with family or friends. In contrast, others may prefer to sit in quiet contemplation.

Recognize that grief does not always follow a linear path. There may be days when the burden seems lighter, and sorting through belongings feels like a celebration of life rather than a reminder of loss. On other days, the sorrow may feel overwhelming. Be patient with yourself and understand that this is a normal part of the emotional journey.

While coping with loss and grief, there is also an opportunity for growth and understanding. By letting go, we can come to terms with our past, reconcile with our present, and make peace with the inevitability of change. Though fraught with emotional challenges, this journey can ultimately lead to a place of acceptance and serenity.

In our lives, it is essential to find balance. Allow grief its time, but also seek out the moments of lightness and joy that can emerge from releasing the old and making space for new experiences. In the next section, we will explore how the act of letting go can be not only a process of decluttering but also a gratifying act of self-discovery and renewal.

Finding Joy in Letting Go

Letting go is a release of the past, clearing space for the future. This journey can lead to unexpected joy and a deep sense of liberation.

As we sift through the layers of belongings, we often stumble upon items that have been long forgotten, tucked away in the corners of drawers or the back of closets. These rediscovered treasures can evoke a complex array of memories, some tinged with nostalgia, others with regret. It is natural to feel a reluctance to part with these objects, as they seem to be tangible links to the experiences and people that have shaped us.

However, a subtle but powerful joy emerges when we give ourselves permission to let go. When we engage in the act of discarding or donating, we not only gain satisfaction, but also recognise that in doing so, we are honoring our past while making room for new experiences. We are not erasing memories but acknowledging that they exist within us, independent of the physical objects that may trigger them.

The joy in letting go also comes from the understanding that our possessions can have a second life that extends beyond our own. By passing on items to family, friends, or even strangers, we allow our belongings to serve a new purpose, to bring happiness or utility to others. This generosity can be incredibly fulfilling, as it connects us to a larger community and contributes to a cycle of giving that has meaningful implications.

The process of letting go can be an opportunity for self-discovery. As we evaluate what to keep and what to release, we are prompted to reflect on what truly matters to us. This introspection can lead to a clearer sense of our values and priorities and influence how we live our lives moving forward. The space we create by decluttering can be both literal and figurative, allowing us to breathe more freely and focus on the aspects of life that bring us the most joy.

In embracing the concept of finding joy in letting go, we also embrace a form of mindfulness. It is a practice that requires us to be present in the moment, engage with our emotions, and make conscious decisions about what we choose to surround ourselves with. This mindfulness can extend to other areas of our lives, encouraging us to live more intentionally and to appreciate the present.

The emotional journey of Swedish death cleaning is not without its challenges. Still, it is a path that can lead to a lighter, more joyful existence. As we learn to let go, we open ourselves up to new possibilities and affirm that our happiness is not bound by the material world but a reflection of the love, relationships, and experiences that truly define us.

The Role of Reflection and Mindfulness

Throughout the pages of this book, we have come to understand that decluttering is far more than a mere physical task; it is a profoundly emotional and reflective journey. As we sift through the layers of our material possessions, we are also sifting through the layers of our lives, memories, and the very essence of our being. This is where the role of reflection and mindfulness becomes paramount.

Reflection, in the context of Swedish death cleaning, is the deliberate act of contemplating the significance of each item in our possession. It is about asking ourselves why we have held onto particular objects and whether they continue to serve a purpose in our lives or those we will one day leave behind. This introspective approach allows us to make decisions not out of haste or obligation but from a place of conscious choice.

On the other hand, mindfulness is the practice of being fully present in the moment and aware of our thoughts and feelings without judgment. As we engage in decluttering, mindfulness keeps us centered and grounded. It helps us to recognize the emotional responses that arise—be it joy, sadness, or nostalgia—and to honor those feelings without becoming overwhelmed by them.

Reflection and mindfulness create a space for us to engage with our belongings thoughtfully and intentionally. By being reflective, we permit ourselves to acknowledge the past, the memories associated with our possessions, and their roles in our lives. By being mindful, we stay connected to the present, ensuring that our actions align with our current values and the legacy we wish to leave.

This process is an opportunity to reassess what we truly value, simplify our lives, and make peace with the impermanence of all things. In embracing reflection and mindfulness, we not only prepare our homes for a future without us, but we also cultivate a sense of peace and fulfillment in the here and now, knowing that we are living—and leaving—a life that is both intentional and meaningful.

Chapter Summary

- Swedish death cleaning involves emotional challenges as one sorts through a lifetime of possessions, evoking memories and feelings.
- The practice is not just about decluttering but also about confronting mortality and the impermanence of life.
- The process can bring joy from rediscovering cherished items but also sadness from parting with objects tied to one's identity.
- Letting go of items can feel like an erasure of life chapters, requiring compassion and patience to handle the emotional lows.
- Deciding what to keep or discard is empowering, helping to reaffirm values and shape one's legacy. It's a reflective journey, prompting questions about the importance of possessions and their role in defining identity.
- Coping with loss and grief is part of the process, with some days feeling lighter and others more sorrowful.
- Finding joy in letting go can lead to liberation, self-discovery, and a more intentional life, unburdened by unnecessary items.

7

PRACTICAL MATTERS

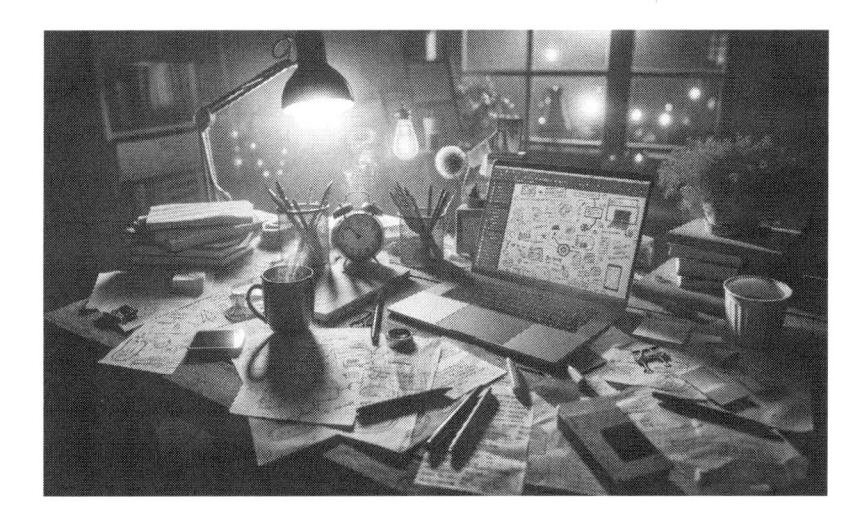

I n this section of the book, we will focus on how to handle legal documents and financial affairs. This is a cornerstone of ensuring that our affairs are in order, both for our peace of mind and to ease the burden on those we leave behind.

Begin with gathering all relevant legal documents. These may include wills, trusts, deeds, and titles. It is essential to keep these documents up to date and in a secure yet accessible location.

Inform a trusted family member or friend about where these documents can be found. If you have appointed an executor for your estate, ensure that this individual knows their responsibilities and the location of these critical documents.

Next, consider your financial affairs. Compile a comprehensive list of bank accounts, investments, insurance policies, and outstanding debts. This list should include institution names, account numbers, and contact information for each entity. It is also wise to include a summary of your regular bills and subscriptions, as these will need to be managed or canceled accordingly.

Reflect on the importance of transparency in these matters. It is not uncommon to feel a sense of privacy about one's finances. However, in the context of death cleaning, openness can prevent unnecessary complications during an already challenging time. Consider writing a letter of instruction that goes beyond the legal formality of a will. This letter can guide your loved ones on how you wish your affairs to be handled and can include personal sentiments and explanations that legal documents may not convey.

As you organize these elements, consider any safe deposit boxes, storage units, and physical items of significant monetary or sentimental value. Document these and communicate their existence and your intentions for them.

In this process, it is advisable to consult with a legal professional to ensure that all documents are in order and that your wishes are articulated and legally sound. This step can prevent disputes and confusion, allowing your loved ones to focus on honoring your memory rather than deciphering legal complexities.

As we conclude this section on legal documents and financial affairs, we pave the way for the next step in Swedish death cleaning: addressing digital assets and passwords. In our modern age, these elements have become integral to our daily lives and, consequently, to the legacy we leave behind.

Addressing Digital Assets and Passwords

Our lives are increasingly intertwined with the digital world in the modern era. As we consider the practical matters of decluttering and organizing our lives, we must pay due attention to our digital assets and passwords. This aspect of death cleaning is about ensuring that our digital legacy is handled with the same care and respect as our physical possessions. We discussed the handling of digital memories in earlier chapters, but this section will explore digital assets in more detail.

Digital assets encompass various elements, from social media accounts and email to online banking and investment portfolios. They also include personal items such as digital photos, videos, and documents often stored in cloud services or various devices. Managing these assets is a two-fold process: first, identifying them, and second, ensuring that loved ones can access them when the time comes.

Begin by creating a comprehensive inventory of your digital assets. This list should include all online accounts and the corresponding usernames and passwords. It's important to keep this inventory updated and to store it securely. Several methods exist to manage this sensitive information, including password managers, encrypted digital storage, or a physical document kept in a safe or with a trusted individual.

Consider how you would like each account handled when documenting your digital assets. Some platforms have policies in place for the accounts of deceased users, and you may have the option to select a legacy contact or set up an account to be memorialized. For other accounts, you may wish to provide instructions on whether they should be deleted, archived, or transferred to someone else.

It's also crucial to understand the legal implications of transferring digital assets. Laws regarding digital property after death may evolve, and it's wise to consult with an attorney to ensure that your wishes are enforceable and that you're adhering to the terms of service agreements for each platform.

Lastly, consider the security of your digital assets. Securely store your passwords, access codes, and any other necessary information so that a trusted individual can access them when the time comes. Digital legacy services and password managers are designed for this purpose, which can simplify the process for your loved ones.

Remember to review and address your digital assets periodically. As technology changes and new platforms emerge, revisit your inventory regularly to add new accounts and remove those no longer active. Communicate with your loved ones about your digital estate plan so they know your wishes and where to find the necessary information when needed.

Incorporating digital assets into your Swedish death cleaning process is a thoughtful way to ease the burden on your loved ones and protect your digital legacy. By taking these methodical steps, you can ensure that your online presence is managed with the same dignity and intention as the rest of your estate.

Estate Planning and Wills

Estate planning and drafting wills are critical components of the death cleaning process, ensuring that our material possessions and assets are distributed according to our wishes upon our departure from this world.

Estate planning is not just a task for older people or the wealthy; it is a practical step for anyone who wishes to have a say in handling their affairs after they are gone. It involves a clear and legally binding document, typically known as a will, which outlines the distribution of one's assets and the care of any dependents. This document serves as a voice that speaks on your behalf, providing instructions and decisions that must be respected and followed.

When engaging in estate planning, it is wise to begin by taking a comprehensive inventory of your assets. These include real estate, bank accounts, investments, insurance policies, and personal items of value such as jewelry, art, or heirlooms. Once the inventory is complete, consider the beneficiaries who will receive parts of your estate. They could be family members, friends, or charitable organizations you wish to support.

Selecting an executor, a trusted individual responsible for carrying out the instructions in your will, is also crucial. This role requires a person who is both willing and able to handle the legal and financial responsibilities that come with the distribution of an estate. It is a role of great trust and should be considered carefully.

In addition to the distribution of assets, a will can include the designation of guardians for minor children, instructions for the continuation or dissolution of a business, and even the care of pets. These personal preferences make your will a unique and personal document, reflecting your assets, values, and wishes.

While the process may seem daunting, numerous resources are available to assist in estate planning. Legal professionals specializing in wills and estates can provide invaluable guidance, ensuring that your will is comprehensive and compliant with current laws. There are also do-it-yourself kits and software for those with straightforward estates. However, professional advice is always recommended to avoid oversights or legal complications.

Once your will is drafted, it is not a document to be tucked away and forgotten. Life's circumstances change, and so too should your will. Regular reviews and updates are necessary to ensure that it accurately reflects your wishes. Major life events such as marriage, divorce, the birth of a child, or the acquisition of significant assets are all reasons to revisit your will.

In the spirit of Swedish death cleaning, estate planning and wills are not about dwelling on the end of life but rather about ensuring peace of mind for yourself and your loved ones. It is an act of kindness and consideration, a way to ease the burden on those who remain and to leave an orderly and transparent legacy.

We will now shift our focus from the tangible aspects of our estate to the more personal and intimate considerations of our final wishes. This naturally leads us to contemplate our funeral wishes and advanced directives, which will be explored in the following section.

Funeral Wishes and Advanced Directives

In the process of Swedish death cleaning, there is a component that often goes unaddressed until it is too late: the articulation of funeral wishes and the creation of advanced directives. You don't have to wait until the later years of your life to consider these aspects. This section will guide you through the thoughtful process of making and documenting these crucial decisions properly.

Funeral wishes can vary widely from individual to individual. Some may desire a traditional burial, while others prefer cremation followed by a memorial service. Some wish for their remains to be scattered in a place of significance, and others opt for newer methods, such as green burials. The key is to reflect on what would be most meaningful to you and your family and to make these wishes known.

Begin by contemplating the type of service you would like. Consider the music, readings, or any specific rituals that hold personal significance. Think about who you would want to speak or perform at the service. These details can offer comfort and a sense of closeness to your loved ones as they carry out your final wishes.

Once you have a clear idea of your preferences, it is crucial to document them. A written plan can be kept with your important papers, such as your will or estate plan, and should be accessible to your next of kin or executor. While this document does not carry the legal weight of a will, it serves as a guide to your loved ones and helps to ensure your wishes are respected.

Advanced directives, on the other hand, are legally binding documents that outline your medical care preferences if you cannot communicate them yourself. These include living wills and health care proxies or durable powers of attorney for health care. A living will details the types of medical treatments you would or would not want to receive in various scenarios, while a health care proxy appoints someone to make medical decisions on your behalf.

Discussing your thoughts and decisions with the person you intend to name as your healthcare proxy is advisable. This conversation can be challenging, but they must understand your values and desires regarding end-of-life care. Additionally, ensure that your healthcare providers have copies of these documents and that they are included in your medical records.

By taking the time to address these matters, you gain peace of mind and provide clarity and direction to those managing your affairs. This foresight is a final act of kindness that relieves your loved ones of the burden of guesswork during a time of grief.

Addressing funeral wishes and advanced directives is a continuation of the thoughtful consideration for the well-being of those we leave behind. It is a way to maintain control over our final narrative and impart a sense of order and calm when needed.

Communicating Your Plans Clearly

Clear communication is important throughout this process. It is a task that requires introspection and the ability to convey your intentions and decisions to those affected by them. After addressing the sensitive topics of funeral wishes and advanced directives, it is essential to pivot towards the broader scope of your plans and how to share them effectively.

To begin, consider creating a comprehensive document that outlines the specifics of your death cleaning process. This document should guide your loved ones, detailing what you have done, why you have made certain choices, and where important items are located. Transparency is vital; the more your family understands your rationale, the easier it will be for them to respect and carry out your wishes.

When communicating your plans, it's essential to be as detailed as possible. For instance, if you have earmarked particular possessions for specific individuals, make a list that matches items with their intended recipients. This will help to prevent misunderstandings and disputes among family members when you are no longer around. If you have decided to donate specific items to charity or sell them, provide instructions on how this should be done, perhaps even suggesting specific organizations that align with your values.

Discussing your plans with your loved ones can be difficult, but it is necessary to ensure that your wishes are understood and respected. Approach the topic with sensitivity and allow for an open dialogue. Your family members may have questions or emotions they need to express, and a face-to-face discussion can provide the clarity and comfort they need.

In addition to verbal communication, consider appointing a trusted executor for your death cleaning plan. This person should be organized, reliable, and willing to take on the responsibility of ensuring your wishes are fulfilled. Provide them with all the necessary documentation and information they will need to fulfill their role effectively.

Remember that the goal of Swedish death cleaning is not only to ease your burden but also to simplify the lives of those you leave behind. By communicating your plans clearly, you create a path for a smoother transition and a loving legacy that reflects your thoughtfulness and consideration.

Chapter Summary

- An essential aspect of Swedish death cleaning involves organizing legal documents and financial affairs for ease of loved ones.
- Gather and update critical legal documents like wills and trusts, informing executors and trusted individuals of their location.
- Compile a list of financial accounts, investments, insurance policies, and debts, including contact information and account details.
- Write a letter of instruction to accompany the will, providing personal guidance and sentiments.
- Document and communicate about safe deposit boxes, storage units, and valuable items.
- Consult a legal professional to ensure documents are legally sound and wishes are clear.
- Address digital assets and passwords by creating an inventory and providing access instructions.
- Estate planning and wills are essential for everyone, not just older people or the wealthy, to distribute assets and care for dependents according to one's wishes.

8

THE ART OF GIVING

In Swedish death cleaning, gift-giving becomes a thoughtful process of transferring memories and affection. As we sort through our possessions, we often come across items that may hold significant value for our loved ones while no longer serving us. This is where gift-giving intertwines with the systematic approach of death cleaning.

Ultimately, the gifts we choose to give as part of our death cleaning should be extensions of our affection and reflect our understanding of the recipient. They are tokens of our legacy, small pieces of ourselves that we entrust to others, hoping to add to their lives the richness of shared moments and lasting memories.

Choosing Meaningful Gifts for Loved Ones

Selecting gifts for our loved ones is both a gesture of affection and an expression of our legacy. To choose these gifts with intention, reflect on the relationships that have shaped our lives. Consider the individual you are gifting to: their interests, memories with you, and the message you wish to convey through this item. It is not the monetary value that defines the worth of a gift in this context but the emotional significance and the shared connection it represents. A well-chosen gift can evoke shared experiences and express understanding and appreciation.

When selecting an item, ask yourself whether it will bring joy, utility, or a sense of connection to the recipient. An heirloom, for instance, may carry the weight of family history and serve as a cherished keepsake. A book that sparked a lifelong passion, a piece of jewelry worn on a memorable occasion, or even a tool that has served you well can be a vessel for stories and sentiments you wish to pass on.

Consider also the story the item carries. A piece of jewelry may be beautiful, but it becomes truly precious when accompanied by the tale of its origin or the memories that accompanied it. Similarly, a book may hold more than the wisdom within its pages; it might also represent a shared interest or a conversation long past.

Consider the practicality of the item in the context of the recipient's life. An heirloom that requires extensive care or a large piece of furniture may not fit comfortably into their space or lifestyle. Finding a different home for these items to be fully appreciated and utilized may be more considerate. Aim for gifts that integrate seamlessly into the lives of your loved ones rather than becoming a burden. In this way, the essence of Swedish death cleaning is honored, as it seeks to lighten the load of both the giver and the receiver.

It is also important to respect the recipient's space and preferences. Open a dialogue with them to ensure your gift is welcomed and not become a burden. This conversation can be a beautiful opportunity to reminisce and reinforce bonds, making the act of giving itself a cherished memory.

The presentation of the gift can be a meaningful ritual. A handwritten note explaining the item's history and meaning in your life can significantly enhance the value of the gift. It transforms the object from a mere material possession into a narrative, a shared chapter in the story of your life and theirs.

Giving these carefully chosen items celebrates life and relationships. It is an opportunity to reflect on the bonds that have sustained us and to offer a piece of ourselves to those who will continue the story long after we are gone. Through these meaningful gifts, we can not only declutter our physical space but also enrich our emotional connection with loved ones.

Donations: Finding the Right Homes for Your Items

Donation is a meaningful and satisfying part of the death cleaning process. Donating our possessions is a way to extend their life beyond our own, to pass on the utility of the items, and to experience the spirit of generosity that comes with giving. It is essential, however, to approach this task with the same level of thoughtfulness we have applied to the rest of our cleaning.

To begin, take stock of the items you wish to donate. These could range from clothing and books to furniture and household goods. Consider the condition of each item. Donations should be in good repair, clean, and presentable. Remember, the goal is to provide something of value, not to offload the responsibility of disposal onto others.

Once you have a clear idea of what you wish to give away, the next step is to find suitable homes for your items. Research local charities and non-profit organizations that accept donations. Many organizations have specific needs or guidelines for what they can accept, so it is important to respect these requirements to ensure your items will be suitable.

Consider the potential impact of your donations. For example, donating professional attire to organizations that help individuals prepare for job interviews can significantly impact someone's life. Books can find new readers through libraries or schools, and furniture can furnish the homes of those in need.

Sometimes, you may wish to donate to specialized programs or causes close to your heart. You may have tools that could benefit a local community workshop or musical instruments that could support a school's arts program. By matching your items with the right recipients, you ensure they are appreciated and support the causes you believe in.

It's also worth considering donating to thrift stores run by charitable organizations. The proceeds from the sale of your items can support various programs and services, multiplying your contribution's impact.

When you have identified where to donate your items, organize them accordingly. Some organizations offer pick-up services; others require you to drop off your donations. Make sure to follow their processes, as this helps maintain the efficiency and effectiveness of their operations.

The act of donating should not be rushed. Take the time to reflect on the potential joy and assistance your items can bring to others. This reflection honors the spirit of döstädning and reinforces the cycle of giving and receiving that enriches our communities.

Finding the right homes for your items transforms your act of decluttering into a gesture of kindness and compassion. Through this process, we can leave a positive imprint on the world, one that resonates with the values we hold dear and the legacy we wish to leave behind.

The Impact of Your Generosity

When you choose to part with your possessions, you are both emptying space in your home and filling spaces in the lives of others. This transition of belongings from one life to another is both a physical handover and a transfer of care, respect, and generosity. Your generosity has a ripple effect that extends far beyond the initial act of giving. It touches lives in ways that are often unseen and unmeasured but deeply felt.

Consider the books that once lined your shelves, offering knowledge, escape, and comfort. In a new reader's hands, they become a source of inspiration, a catalyst for education, or a companion in solitude. The clothes you once wore, each thread woven with memories, now provide warmth and dignity to someone who may have stood vulnerable against the elements. The toys that echoed with the laughter of your children can now bring joy to another child's heart, enabling them to create their own cherished memories.

Your act of giving does not end with the physical transfer of items. It plants seeds of kindness that may bloom in unexpected ways. The recipients of your belongings may be moved to continue the cycle of generosity, passing on the items they received from you and the spirit in which they were given. In this way, your influence extends into the community, fostering a culture of giving and sharing.

The process of letting go is also a gift to yourself. It is an opportunity to reflect on what truly matters in life and to cherish the memories associated with your possessions without being anchored by them. It allows you to make peace with the impermanence of material things and to focus on the enduring nature of relationships and experiences.

The impact of your generosity is both intimate and expansive. It demonstrates the interconnectedness of our lives and the shared humanity that binds us. Through giving, you contribute to a legacy of kindness that will outlive the physical presence of the items you have parted with.

Gratitude and Reciprocity

The act of giving is a two-way street. It is a path paved with gratitude and reciprocity that enriches the experience for both the giver and the receiver. As we bestow our belongings to others, it helps to understand the raw exchange of emotions and values that occurs in this process.

Gratitude, in its purest form, is the recognition of the kindness that others have shown us. When we give away our possessions, particularly those with sentimental value, we share a piece of our life's narrative. The recipients of these items often feel a deep appreciation for the physical gift and the trust and affection it symbolizes. This gratitude is a powerful force, capable of deepening bonds and creating lasting memories.

Reciprocity, on the other hand, is the response to the gratitude felt. It is an innate human instinct to want to return kindness when it is received. Reciprocity may not always manifest in the form of physical items. Sometimes, it is the emotional support offered during the cleaning process, the shared stories about the items being passed on, or the simple act of acknowledging the effort to sort through a lifetime of belongings.

The beauty of this exchange is that it creates a cycle of goodwill that extends beyond the material. As we select items to give away, we invite others to partake in our history, and, in doing so, we also give them the opportunity to contribute to the narrative. They may reciprocate by sharing their own stories, providing companionship, or offering assistance in the practical aspects of the cleaning.

Approach this exchange without expectation, understanding that its value lies in the act itself rather than any potential return. The essence of Swedish death cleaning is to lighten the load of our existence, simplify our spaces and lives, and make our departure less burdensome for others. When we engage in this practice with a heart full of gratitude and an openness to reciprocity, we not only enrich our own lives but also bring warmth and connection to the lives of others.

As we continue to navigate the layers of belongings and memories, do so with the knowledge that each item we part with carries the potential for a meaningful exchange. The gratitude and reciprocity that flow from these acts of giving are the threads that weave the fabric of human connection, making the process of Swedish death cleaning a truly transformative experience.

Chapter Summary

- Gift-giving is a thoughtful way to pass on memories and affection to others.
- Gifts should be chosen for their emotional resonance and connection to the recipient, not monetary value.
- Respect the recipient's space and preferences, ensuring the gift is welcomed. Practicality should be considered; items requiring extensive care or space may not be suitable.
- Donating items as part of death cleaning extends their usefulness and embodies generosity. Donations should be in good condition and given to organizations where they will be valued.

- Giving has a ripple effect, fostering a culture of generosity and community support.
- Swedish death cleaning is a reciprocal process, fostering gratitude and deepening human connections.

9

OVERCOMING CHALLENGES

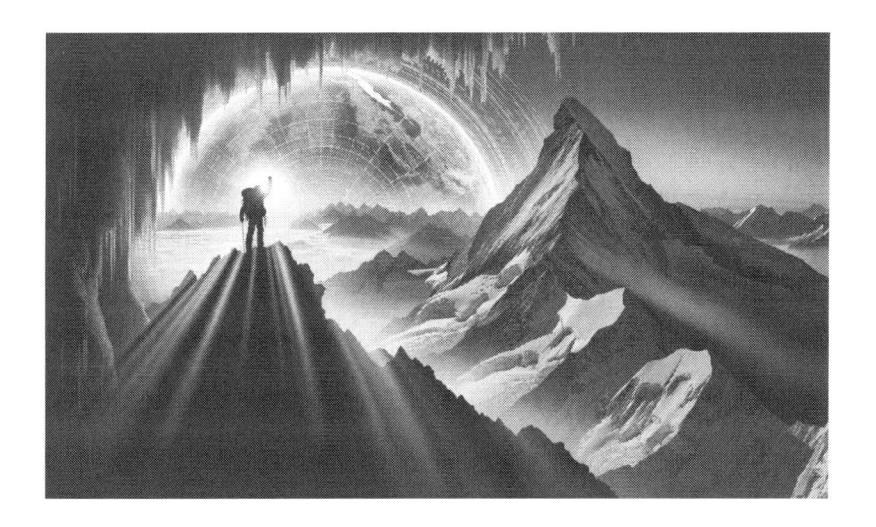

During your journey, you may find yourself face to face with two formidable adversaries: procrastination and overwhelm. These challenges are inherent in sorting through a lifetime's accumulation of possessions, and can be as much a part of the journey as the items themselves.

Procrastination often appears when we are confronted with tasks that seem monumental in scope. The thought of sorting through decades of belongings can be daunting, leading to a paralysis of action. It is a natural response to an overwhelming task that can be overcome with small steps and a shift in perspective.

Break the task into manageable segments to combat procrastination. Start with a single drawer, a particular category of items, or a defined space within your home. Compartmentalizing the process makes the task less intimidating, and each small victory can propel you forward. Setting aside regular, scheduled times for death cleaning can also create a routine that helps overcome the inertia that procrastination breeds.

Overwhelm, on the other hand, can engulf us when the emotional weight of our possessions comes to bear. Each object may hold a memory, sentiment, or piece of our past. The key to navigating this emotional landscape is acknowledging and permitting yourself to experience all the feelings that arise. Reflect on the significance of each item and the freedom and peace that will come from letting go.

It is also helpful to remember why you chose to do this in the first place. Was it to ease the burden on loved ones, curate a collection of items that reflect your life, or to declutter your living space and mind? Focusing on the benefits the process will bring makes it easier to push through the emotional and physical work involved.

Overwhelm can also stem from the sheer volume of items to sort through. In such cases, enlisting help from friends, family, or professionals can provide practical and emotional assistance. Sharing stories and memories as you sort through items can transform the process from a solitary chore into a shared experience, enriching the process and dispersing the weight of decision-making.

Ultimately, the journey through procrastination and feeling overwhelmed is part of the journey and requires patience and self-compassion. It is a process of revisiting the past, confronting the present, and preparing for the future. By approaching it with a reflective mindset and a systematic plan, the path becomes clearer, and the task is more approachable. With each item released, space is created—not just in the home, but in the heart and mind—for new experiences and a sense of tranquility that comes with knowing your legacy will be a blessing, not a burden.

Dealing with Resistance from Others

As you declutter your belongings, you may find that the challenge is not solely within yourself but also resistance from those around you—family, friends, and loved ones who may not immediately understand or support this process.

Resistance from others can manifest in various ways. It may come as a surprise when a family member expresses a strong emotional attachment to an item you are ready to part with, or when a friend questions the necessity of this practice, labeling it as morbid or unnecessary. These reactions are rooted in personal connections to the objects in question or from a discomfort with the concept of mortality that Swedish death cleaning inherently acknowledges.

To navigate this resistance, approach these conversations with empathy and patience. Begin by explaining the purpose and benefits of Swedish death cleaning—for yourself and those around you. Emphasize that this process is not about erasing memories but curating them, ensuring that the most significant and meaningful items are preserved without clutter.

When facing emotional attachments from others, listen and acknowledge their feelings. Engage in dialogue about the memories associated with the items and consider if there are alternative ways to honor them, such as through photographs or shared stories, rather than the physical possession itself.

In instances where resistance stems from a discomfort with the concept of death, it may be helpful to reframe the conversation around simplification and mindfulness in your current life. Swedish death cleaning is as much about living a more organized and intentional life now as it is about preparing for the future.

Setting boundaries and asserting your autonomy in the process is also beneficial. While it is important to consider the feelings of others, ultimately, the decision of what to keep and what to let go of is personal. You should gently remind others that while their input is valued, the final choices are yours.

Involving family and friends in the process can sometimes turn resistance into support. Invite them to participate in sorting through items, sharing stories, and making decisions about family heirlooms. This inclusive approach can transform the process into a collective journey, fostering understanding and inspiring others to consider their relationship with possessions.

Lastly, remember to maintain perspective. Resistance from others is often a reflection of their internal struggles and not a rejection of your efforts. You may gradually influence their perceptions and alleviate their concerns by demonstrating the positive changes and the sense of peace from Swedish death cleaning.

In the following section, we will explore how to address the physical limitations that may arise during Swedish death cleaning and the importance of seeking and accepting help when needed.

Physical Limitations and Asking for Help

Choosing to embark on the journey of Swedish death cleaning is a testament to your courage and commitment to mindful living. However, physical limitations can sometimes present significant hurdles in this process. Sorting, lifting, and organizing one's possessions can be demanding. For some, these tasks might be challenging or unfeasible due to age, health, or disability.

It is at this point that asking for help becomes necessary. The ethos of Swedish death cleaning is not to burden others with one's belongings after you pass on. Similarly, it should not burden the individual undertaking it in the present. Seeking assistance is a practical step that aligns with the spirit of the process.

When physical constraints impede your ability to carry out specific tasks, consider contacting family, friends, or professional services. This support network can provide the physical strength and endurance the task demands.

Communicate your needs and intentions clearly when asking for help. Be specific about the assistance you require, whether sorting through heavy boxes, rearranging furniture, or deciding about particular items. Those who care for you will likely appreciate the opportunity to contribute to your well-being, and the peace of mind of knowing your affairs are in order.

Respecting the boundaries and limitations of those you ask for help is equally important. Be mindful of their time and physical capabilities, and express gratitude for their assistance. If necessary, consider hiring professional help, such as a home organizer or a moving service, which can provide expertise and efficiency.

In instances where help is not readily available, it may be wise to approach the task incrementally. Break down the process into smaller, manageable tasks that align with your physical capacity. This approach not only respects your limitations but also ensures steady progress.

Swedish death cleaning is not a race against time but a thoughtful progression towards simplicity and order. It is about making the process as gentle and kind to oneself as it is to others. By acknowledging the need for help and embracing it, you honor the essence of this practice—reducing the burden on oneself and others and paving the way for a legacy of care and consideration.

Staying Motivated and Keeping Momentum

Döstädning is a process of reflection and a journey towards a tidier, more intentional living space. However, as with any journey, maintaining the drive to continue is crucial. This section will explore strategies to stay motivated and keep momentum during the decluttering process.

Firstly, set clear, achievable goals. Sorting through your possessions can be daunting, so breaking it down into smaller, more manageable tasks can make the process feel less overwhelming. Consider setting aside specific times for cleaning, perhaps an hour each day or a few hours on the weekend, and focus on one area at a time. Completing these mini-goals can provide a sense of accomplishment and encourage you to continue.

Another way to maintain motivation is to keep in mind the reasons why you started this process. Reflect on the benefits that Swedish death cleaning can bring, not only to you but also to your loved ones. The peace of mind that comes from knowing you are not leaving a burden for others can be a powerful motivator. Additionally, the act of decluttering can be liberating and can lead to a more serene living environment.

Visual progress is another motivator. Before you start, take photographs of the areas you plan to declutter. As you make progress, take new photos to document the transformation. Seeing the physical change in your space can be incredibly satisfying and spur you to continue.

Reward yourself for milestones reached. After completing a particularly challenging area, treat yourself to something enjoyable: a nice meal, a relaxing bath, or an evening with a good book. These rewards can serve as incentives to push through the more challenging parts of the cleaning process.

Finally, be patient with yourself. There will be days when

progress is slow, which is perfectly acceptable. The key is to keep moving forward, even one small step at a time.

By implementing these strategies, you can maintain motivation and momentum throughout your Swedish death cleaning journey. Each can help transform what may seem impossible into a fulfilling and life-affirming process.

Adapting the Process to Fit Your Needs

Now, let us turn our attention to the personalization of döstädning to meet your own personal needs. This process is not a one-size-fits-all endeavor; it is an intricate and individualized journey that requires adaptation to circumstances and needs.

Your life is unique, and so is your home. Your memories, possessions, and emotional attachments are yours alone. Therefore, the sorting and decluttering process should be tailored to reflect your individuality. You should craft a method that resonates with your lifestyle, values, and goals.

Begin by assessing your living space and belongings with a discerning eye. Consider the size of your home, the number of items you possess, and your physical ability to manage the task at hand. If you live in a large house with decades' worth of belongings, your approach will differ from someone in a smaller apartment. Similarly, you may need to pace yourself differently or seek assistance if you have physical limitations.

Consider your emotional readiness. Swedish death cleaning is also about confronting the emotional weight of your possessions. Some items may be easy to part with, while others may require more reflection and time. Allow yourself the flexibility to handle these items at your own pace, perhaps revisiting them after you've gained momentum with less sentimental objects.

Furthermore, your method of disposal should align with your

values. If environmental concerns are important to you, seek ways to recycle or donate items rather than discard them. If you wish to leave a legacy, consider which items might be meaningful to pass on to family members or friends and have conversations with them about these pieces.

Incorporate elements of Swedish death cleaning into your routine in a manageable way—whether that means dedicating a set amount of time each day or week to the task or integrating it into your regular cleaning schedule.

Be kind to yourself during this process. There will be moments of doubt and hesitation, but also times of clarity and liberation. By adapting the principles and strategies we've explored to fit your needs and circumstances, you create a more manageable and meaningful path for you.

Chapter Summary

- Swedish death cleaning is a decluttering process that involves emotional release and can be hindered by procrastination and overwhelm.
- Break the task into smaller segments to combat procrastination and schedule regular cleaning times.
- Overwhelm can be managed by acknowledging emotions tied to possessions and focusing on the benefits of decluttering for oneself and loved ones.
- Enlisting help from friends, family, or professionals can provide practical and emotional support during the process.
- Resistance from others may occur; approach these situations with empathy, patience, and clear communication about the purpose of death cleaning.

- Physical limitations may require asking for help from others or hiring professional services to assist with the cleaning process.
- Staying motivated involves setting clear goals, involving others, documenting progress, rewarding oneself, and being patient.
- The cleaning process should be personalized to fit your needs, considering your living space, physical ability, emotional readiness, and values.

10

LIFE AFTER DEATH CLEANING

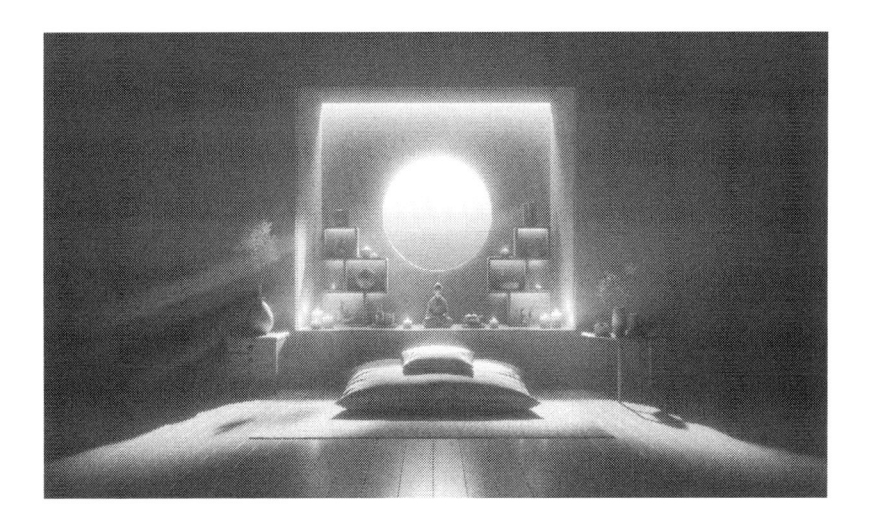

We have traversed through the philosophical underpinnings and the practical steps of decluttering your life in preparation to create a simpler, clutter-free future. It is now time to reflect on the transformative impact this process can have on our day-to-day existence. Reducing our possessions involves a conscious choice to embrace a minimalist lifestyle.

At its core, minimalism is about paring down life to its essentials. It is a deliberate decision to eschew the material in favor of what truly adds value to our lives. In Swedish death cleaning, minimalism takes on a poignant significance. It is about creating a serene environment that reflects our most cherished values, making room for the activities and relationships that enrich our existence.

The freedom that comes with living with less is multifaceted. Fewer possessions mean less time and energy spent on cleaning, maintenance, and organization. This newfound time can be redirected towards hobbies, passions, or simply the joy of leisure. It is a liberation from the relentless pursuit of material acquisitions that often defines modern life.

Physically, the spaces we inhabit become more open and tranquil. There is a tangible peace that comes with the absence of excess. Rooms are easier to navigate, clean, and maintain, saving time and reducing the stress associated with household chores. This simplicity in our surroundings can lead to a more serene lifestyle, where the emphasis is on living, not maintaining possessions.

Psychologically, the benefits are equally far-reaching. A minimalist lifestyle can lead to a clearer mind, reduced anxiety, and a greater sense of control. In the absence of clutter, there is space for clarity and focus. The mind, no longer preoccupied with the chaos of clutter, can focus more readily on the present moment, fostering a state of mindfulness often elusive in a world of material distractions. The things we keep around us gain greater significance, and we become more mindful of what we allow into our personal space.

Emotionally, the freedom of living with less can be liberating. The ties to the past, often embodied in the form of material goods, can be gently severed, allowing for a forward-looking perspective. This is not to say that all memories or sentimental items are discarded, but rather that a selective process helps to prioritize what truly matters. The emotional weight of objects is acknowledged, but it no longer anchors us to a bygone era.

Embracing minimalism can also have a positive impact on our relationships. We can foster deeper connections with our loved ones with fewer distractions and less emphasis on material wealth. It encourages us to value experiences over objects, creating memories that outlast any physical item.

Financially, the minimalist approach Swedish death cleaning advocates can lead to a more sustainable way of living. Buying less and choosing quality over quantity can reduce our ecological footprint and contribute to a more ethical consumer culture. The savings accrued from this lifestyle can be allocated to more meaningful pursuits or set aside for future security.

Swedish death cleaning is not a singular event, but a continuous practice that encourages us to evaluate our belongings and our attachment to them regularly. This ongoing process helps to cultivate a sense of detachment from material goods, reinforcing the idea that our worth is not measured by what we own but by the richness of our experiences and relationships.

The benefits of living with less extend beyond the individual to the communal and environmental levels. By consuming and hoarding less, we contribute to a culture of sustainability that values resources and reduces the ecological footprint left behind for future generations. It is a conscious choice to partake in a lifestyle that respects the finite nature of our planet's resources.

The minimalist lifestyle that emerges from Swedish death cleaning is about making intentional choices. It is a commitment to live with purpose and to recognize that our possessions do not define us. As we continue to explore the implications of this transformative cleaning process, it becomes clear that letting go involves more than just preparing for our departure from this world. It is also about enhancing the quality of our lives while we are here, creating a legacy of simplicity and intentionality.

In embracing the freedom of living with less, we find that our lives are not diminished but enhanced. The space we create by letting go of the unnecessary allows for new experiences, relationships, and opportunities to enter. It is a space that breathes, grows, and adapts with us as we continue our journey through life, ever mindful of the legacy we wish to leave behind.

Continuing the Practices of Döstädning

Embracing the principles of döstädning is a transformative lifestyle choice that extends beyond the initial clutter purge. This philosophy, rooted in practicality and mindfulness, encourages a continuous cycle of evaluating the necessity and emotional value of our possessions. By integrating the practices of döstädning into our daily lives, we not only prepare for the eventual ease of our passing but also cultivate an environment that reflects a life of intention and clarity.

To continue the practices of döstädning, one must adopt a reflective approach to consumption and possession. This means regularly assessing items for their current utility and emotional significance. The question, "Will anyone I know be happier if I save this?" becomes a guiding mantra, prompting thoughtful decision-making. It's about recognizing that our belongings have a lifecycle, much like ourselves, and being at peace with letting go when the time is right.

An organized system is also key to maintaining the principles of döstädning. This involves setting aside time, perhaps seasonally or annually, to revisit each space in your home. During these times, you can re-evaluate items that may have slipped back into obscurity, ensuring that everything you own remains purposeful or cherished. It's not about creating a stark or sterile environment but about maintaining a harmonious space filled only with items that serve a positive function in your life.

Keeping your personal documents, accounts, and legal matters in order is an ongoing process that requires regular attention. This ensures that, in the event of one's passing, the practical aspects of dealing with their estate are as straightforward and unburdened by complication as possible.

In this way, the practices of döstädning offer a form of self-care that extends to caring for those we will one day leave behind. It is a thoughtful and continuous process of considering our material legacy and the impact it will have on our loved ones. By choosing to live with less and being intentional about what we keep in our lives, we free ourselves from the physical weight of unnecessary possessions and the mental and emotional burdens they can represent.

As we journey through life, embracing the simplicity and foresight that döstädning provides, we find that the benefits of this practice are not confined to the end of life. The peace of mind and freedom that come from a decluttered and well-ordered environment enhance our daily existence, allowing us to live more fully in the present while thoughtfully preparing for the future.

Sharing Your Experience and Inspiring Others

As you continue on the transformative journey of Swedish death cleaning, you may find that the impact of this practice extends far beyond the confines of your own home and personal space. The process of mindfully decluttering and organizing your possessions in anticipation of life's final chapter is not only a gift to yourself but also to those who will carry on after you. It is a profound act of love and consideration that can inspire and guide others in their journeys toward simplicity and intentionality.

Sharing your experience of death cleaning with friends, family, and even broader communities can be a powerful way to extend the benefits of this practice. It is not uncommon for individuals who have undergone döstädning to feel a sense of liberation and peace, which can be contagious. When you talk about the emotional relief and clarity that comes from letting go of unnecessary belongings, you may notice a spark of interest or recognition in your listeners' eyes.

Consider how you can communicate your story. You may start with casual conversations, where you can discuss the positive changes you've noticed in your daily life. You could share anecdotes about items that held special memories and how you chose to honor those memories, whether by keeping, gifting, or thoughtfully disposing of those items.

For those more inclined to engage with larger audiences, writing a blog post, hosting a workshop, or even starting a support group could be effective ways to spread the philosophy and practical steps of Swedish death cleaning. In these settings, you can delve deeper into the emotional aspects of the process, the challenges you faced, and the strategies you employed to overcome them.

It's important to approach these discussions with sensitivity and understanding, as death cleaning can evoke many emotions, from apprehension to curiosity. By sharing your own vulnerabilities and learning experiences, you create a safe space for others to explore their feelings and questions about the practice.

Being open about your difficulties and how you addressed them provides a realistic perspective to help others set reasonable expectations for their death cleaning journey. Your unique approach to sorting through belongings, deciding what to keep, and finding new homes for items you no longer need can serve as a blueprint for others.

Remember that your story has the power to motivate change. As people in your circle begin to see the tangible results of your efforts—perhaps a more organized living space, a lighter emotional load, or a renewed sense of purpose—they may be encouraged to embark on their own paths of mindful decluttering.

In sharing your experience, you are not only recounting a personal tale of decluttering and preparation but also imparting a philosophy of living with intention. Swedish death cleaning is as much about examining one's life and values as it is about physical possessions. Inspiring others to consider what is important contributes to a broader cultural shift toward mindfulness and sustainability.

Sharing your experience with Swedish death cleaning is an extension of the practice itself. It is an opportunity to reflect on the journey, to consolidate the lessons learned, and to offer guidance to those who may one day walk a similar path. Your story, woven from practicality, reflection, and systematic planning, will inspire others as they navigate the complexities of their own lives, possessions, and the legacy they wish to leave behind.

The Ongoing Journey of Self-Discovery

Swedish death cleaning is a transformative journey into the heart of who we are, what we value, and how we wish to be remembered. As we declutter the layers of our material possessions, we are often confronted with the layers of our identity, peeling back the years and the memories that have defined us.

Organizing and letting go of our physical belongings can be a very introspective experience. Each object, whether a treasured photograph, a well-worn book, or a seemingly insignificant trinket, holds a mirror up to our lives, reflecting the moments we've lived and the emotions we've felt. In this way, Swedish death cleaning transcends its practical purposes and catalyzes self-discovery.

As we continue on this path, our relationship with our possessions shifts. What once seemed indispensable may now appear redundant. We learn to distinguish between what genuinely enriches our lives and what merely occupies space. This understanding extends beyond the physical realm; it influences our choices, relationships, and sense of purpose. We start to prioritize experiences over objects, quality over quantity, and meaningful connections over fleeting interactions.

This process often prompts us to consider our legacy. What are the stories we want to tell? What wisdom do we hope to impart? And what would we like to leave behind, not just in terms of physical items, but in the memories and impacts we've had on others? It is in this way that Swedish death cleaning also becomes about refining the quality of our living.

In embracing the principles of Swedish death cleaning, we embark on a continuous journey of self-discovery. It is a process that does not end with the last discarded item but evolves with us. With each object we release, we reaffirm our values and vision for the life we desire. In this ongoing practice, we find a sense of preparedness for our eventual departure and a deeper appreciation for the present moment and the transient beauty of life itself.

Chapter Summary

- Swedish death cleaning is a decluttering philosophy that prepares for death and embraces minimalism. Minimalism involves focusing on essentials, valuing experiences over possessions, and creating a serene environment.
- Living with fewer possessions can lead to less time spent on maintenance and more on hobbies and relationships.

- A minimalist lifestyle can reduce anxiety, increase focus, and improve financial sustainability.
- Regularly practicing Swedish death cleaning can help maintain a decluttered space and keep personal affairs in order.
- Sharing experiences of death cleaning can inspire others to adopt a minimalist lifestyle and focus on what's important.
- The process is about physical decluttering, self-discovery, and considering one's legacy.
- Swedish death cleaning is an ongoing journey that enhances the present and prepares for the future.

THE LASTING IMPACT OF SWEDISH DEATH CLEANING

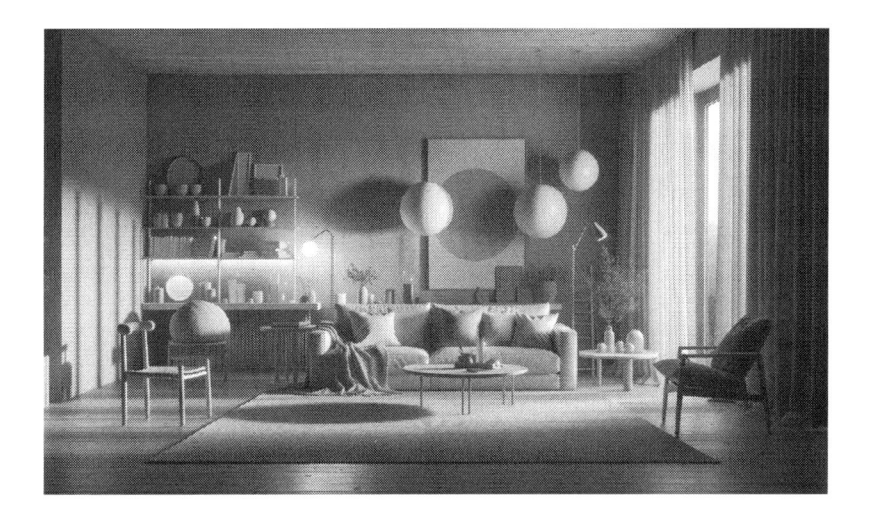

As we approach the conclusion of our exploration into the practice of Swedish death cleaning, let us pause and reflect upon the personal transformation that accompanies this journey. The process, which began as a practical endeavor to declutter and organize one's possessions in preparation for the inevitable, often evolves into a profound exercise in self-discovery and personal growth.

Throughout the chapters of this book, we have discovered the various aspects of Swedish death cleaning, from its pragmatic steps to its emotional nuances. Now, as we stand at the final chapter, it is time to turn our gaze inward and contemplate the internal changes that have taken place.

For many, sorting through a lifetime's worth of belongings extends beyond physical tidiness; it becomes about reconciling one's history. Each object, whether kept, discarded, or passed on, carries a narrative, a fragment of one's identity. Through death cleaning, individuals often encounter forgotten memories, confront unresolved emotions, and reconnect with their past selves. This confrontation with one's life story can lead to a sense of closure and peace as if by organizing our external world, we inadvertently arrange the scattered pieces of our inner world.

Swedish death cleaning prompts us to reevaluate what truly holds value in our lives. As we sift through the material possessions surrounding us, we are compelled to ask ourselves which items serve a purpose and which merely occupy space. This understanding extends beyond the physical realm; it encourages a broader contemplation of our priorities, relationships, and the legacy we wish to leave behind. It is common for many to emerge from this process with a renewed focus on the quality of their connections and experiences rather than the quantity of their possessions.

The introspective nature of death cleaning also fosters a heightened awareness of mortality. While this may initially seem unsettling, it often leads to a more intentional approach to living. Recognizing the impermanence of life can inspire us to make the most of our time, cherish the present, and act with purpose and kindness. The clarity gained from contemplating our finitude can be a powerful catalyst for living a life aligned with our deepest values.

In embracing the principles of Swedish death cleaning, we inadvertently embark on a journey of self-improvement. The lessons learned extend far beyond the confines of our homes and into the essence of our being. As we declutter our physical spaces, we simultaneously clear the way for personal growth, allowing for new experiences, insights, and a deeper understanding of ourselves.

Consider how this personal transformation can ripple outward, influencing not only our own lives but also the lives of those around us. The impact of Swedish death cleaning, as we will explore in the following pages, can reach far beyond the individual, touching the lives of family, friends, and the broader community.

The Ripple Effect on Family and Community

Swedish death cleaning is not merely a solitary act of decluttering or organizing one's possessions in anticipation of life's final chapter. It is a process that extends beyond the individual, touching the lives of everyone around them in lasting ways.

When someone begins the journey of Swedish death cleaning, they are often motivated by the desire to ease the burden on their loved ones after their passing. This thoughtful gesture, however, has a ripple effect that goes beyond the practicalities of minimizing possessions. It can transform relationships as family members engage in conversations about the significance of various items, sharing stories and memories that might otherwise have remained unspoken. These dialogues often lead to a deeper understanding and appreciation of one's heritage and family history, strengthening bonds and fostering a sense of continuity.

Swedish death cleaning can inspire others to reflect on their consumption habits and the accumulation of material goods. As family members witness the benefits of living with less and the peace of mind that comes with a decluttered space, they may be encouraged to embark on their journeys of simplification. This can lead to a collective shift towards more mindful living, focusing on the quality of experiences rather than the quantity of possessions.

The community at large can also benefit from Swedish death cleaning. Items that someone no longer needs or wants can find new life with others who may need them. Donations to local charities, second-hand stores, and community centers extend the usefulness of these items and support the welfare of others within the community. Giving can foster a spirit of generosity and interconnectedness, reminding us that our actions can contribute to the well-being of those around us.

Furthermore, the environmental impact of Swedish death cleaning should not be overlooked. Individuals contribute to a more sustainable way of living by consciously choosing to downsize and recycle. This can lead to a greater awareness of environmental issues within the community and encourage collective efforts to reduce waste and promote responsible consumption.

Swedish death cleaning is more than a method for organizing one's physical belongings; it catalyzes positive change that resonates through families and communities. It prompts us to consider the material legacy we leave behind and the emotional and social imprint we make on the world. It reminds us that the choices we make today can shape the lives of others and the communities we are a part of long after we are gone.

Envisioning Your Legacy

Swedish death cleaning encourages us to envision the mark we want to leave on the world and how we want to be remembered by those who survive us.

Legacy is a tapestry woven from the threads of our actions, choices, and the material echoes we leave behind. Döstädning is a deliberate and thoughtful approach to shaping the narrative of our lives as perceived by future generations. It is about creating a curated collection of our existence that highlights the values and relationships we hold dear.

In paring down our belongings, we can reassess our life's narrative. What are the items that truly matter? Which objects tell the story of who we are and the life we've lived? By keeping what is meaningful, we allow our legacy to shine through the clutter of everyday existence. This is not about erasing our presence but distilling it to its essence, ensuring that what remains reflects our self.

This process is an act of kindness and consideration. It is a way to ease the burden on our loved ones, sparing them the daunting task of sifting through our possessions in a time of grief. It is a final act of care, a way to gently guide them through the remnants of our lives, making mourning and remembrance a little less overwhelming.

Swedish death cleaning is a ritual that helps us confront our mortality with grace and intention, allowing us to leave behind a meaningful and considerate legacy. It is a final gift to those we love, a way to say, "I cared enough to make this easier for you."

As you move forward, carry with you the understanding that the clarity and simplicity you create through this process can serve as a guiding light for your loved ones. It is a way to say farewell with mindfulness and respect, ensuring that our departure is as clean and ordered as the life we strove to lead.

Closing Thoughts and Gratitude

As we conclude our exploration into the thoughtful practice of Swedish death cleaning, it is fitting to pause and reflect on the everlasting effects this tradition can have on our lives and those we leave behind. Decluttering and organizing our possessions with the end in mind is both a practical endeavor and a deeply emotional and spiritual journey that touches the core of our human experience.

Döstädning transcends the simple act of tidying up. It is a deliberate and purposeful way of reviewing one's life, acknowledging the impermanence of our existence, and expressing gratitude for the objects and memories that have accompanied us along the way. Through this lens, each item we choose to pass on or let go of becomes a testament to our lives and our connections.

In practicing Swedish death cleaning, we offer a final gift to our loved ones: the gift of simplicity. By curating our belongings, we alleviate the burden that might otherwise fall on family and friends during a time of grief. This act of service is imbued with love and consideration, ensuring that our departure is not overshadowed by the daunting task of sorting through all of our accumulated belongings.

This process can be a catalyst for expressing gratitude for the myriad experiences that have shaped us. As we sift through our belongings, we can recount our stories, share our history, and impart the wisdom we have gained. This can be an incredibly meaningful exchange between generations, as cherished heirlooms and personal anecdotes are passed down, keeping our legacy alive.

Swedish death cleaning prompts us to live more intentionally in the present. By regularly assessing what we own and why we own it, we become more mindful of our consumption and the footprint we leave behind. This heightened awareness can lead to a more sustainable and purposeful lifestyle that values quality over quantity and experiences over possessions.

In gratitude, we must acknowledge that Swedish death cleaning is not just about preparing for the end. It is about enhancing the quality of our current existence by creating a harmonious and clutter-free environment that allows us to focus on what truly matters. It is about living with intention and leaving with grace.

As we close this chapter, let us embody the lessons of Swedish death cleaning with a sense of peace and preparedness. May we approach the future and the end of our days with the same care and dignity with which we have lived our lives thus far, and may the legacy we leave be as orderly and serene as the spaces we have curated.

ABOUT THE AUTHOR

Hanna Bentsen is an expert in the art of mindful aging and intentional living. With a compassionate voice and a wealth of experience, her work revolutionizes the way we perceive aging and life's inevitable transitions and redefines the middle and later years as periods of growth and enrichment.

Her insightful explorations into Swedish Death Cleaning and the art of aging with grace challenge societal norms, encouraging readers to approach decluttering and aging with intention and dignity. Hanna's books empower readers to embrace the later stages of life with newfound purpose and vitality. They offer practical wisdom for decluttering life's physical and emotional spaces.

Hanna's love for Scandinavian culture, with its emphasis on simplicity and functionality, deeply influences her approach to a well-lived life.